THE BIOCHEMISTRY
OF INTRACELLULAR
PARASITISM

THE SCIENTIST'S LIBRARY
Biology and Medicine

EDITED BY
PETER P. H. DE BRUYN, M.D.

THE BIOCHEMISTRY
OF INTRACELLULAR
PARASITISM

BY

JAMES W. MOULDER

Department of Microbiology
The University of Chicago

THE UNIVERSITY OF CHICAGO PRESS

CHICAGO AND LONDON

THE UNIVERSITY OF CHICAGO COMMITTEE
ON PUBLICATIONS IN BIOLOGY AND MEDICINE

Library of Congress Catalog Card Number: 62-12636

THE UNIVERSITY OF CHICAGO PRESS, CHICAGO 60637
THE UNIVERSITY OF CHICAGO PRESS, LTD., LONDON W.C. 1

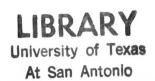

Preface to the Series

During the past few decades the investigative approaches to biological problems have become markedly diversified. This diversification has been caused in part by the introduction of methods from other fields, such as mathematics, physics, and chemistry, and in part has been brought about by the formulation of new problems within biology. At the same time, the quantity of scientific production and publication has increased. Under these circumstances, the biologist has to focus his attention more and more exclusively on his own field of interest. This specialization, effective as it is in the pursuit of individual problems, requiring ability and knowledge didactically unrelated to biology, is detrimental to a broad understanding of the current aspects of biology as a whole, without which conceptual progress is difficult.

The purpose of "The Scientist's Library: Biology and Medicine" series is to provide authoritative information about the growth and status of various subjects in such a fashion that the individual books may be read with profit not only by the specialist but also by those whose interests lie in other fields. The topics for the series have been selected as representative of active fields of science, especially those that have developed markedly in recent years as the result of new methods and new discoveries.

The textual approach is somewhat different from that ordinarily used by the specialist. The authors have been asked to emphasize introductory concepts and problems, and the present status of their subjects, and to clarify terminology and methods of approach instead of limiting themselves to detailed accounts of current factual knowledge. The authors have also been asked to assume a common level of scientific competence rather than to attempt popularization of the subject matter.

Consequently, the books should be of interest and value to workers in the various fields of biology and medicine. For the teacher and investigator, and for students entering specialized areas, they will provide familiarity with the aims, achievements, and present status of these fields.

PETER P. H. DE BRUYN

CHICAGO, ILLINOIS

vi

Foreword

This book examines the contribution of biochemical concepts and techniques to our understanding of the intimate and integrated relationship between a host cell and a parasite growing inside it. The data used for illustration were chosen on the basis of familiarity, availability, and appropriateness. The treatment is not intended to be exhaustive, and many publications in the field have not been discussed—deliberately, when I did not consider them pertinent, and inadvertently, when I did not know about them.

Research in my laboratory has been supported by generous grants from the National Institute of Allergy and Infectious Diseases (United States Public Health Service), the Chemical Corps Biological Laboratories (Fort Detrick), the Abbott Laboratories, the John A. Hartford Foundation, and the Dr. Wallace C. and Clara A. Abbott Memorial Fund of the University of Chicago.

I wish to thank my students and associates who read this book in manuscript; Dr. Martha R. Sheek, who allowed me to read her unpublished doctoral dissertation; and the many authors who permitted me to reproduce electron micrographs from their publications in the illustrations for the book. Dr. Dietrich Peters and Dr. Jack Litwin contributed previously unpublished electron micrographs. I am deeply grateful to Doris Randall for her skill and devotion in preparing the manuscript.

Contents

Illustrations

Illustrations

Diagrams

Tables

CHAPTER I

The Common Feast

. . . biology teaches us that parasitism is a normal phenomenon. . . .

THEOBALD SMITH

parasite (par′à·sĭt), n. [F. fr. L. *parasitus* fr. Gr. *parasitos*, lit., eating beside, or at the table of another, fr. *para* beside + *sitos* food]. **1.** *Gr. Antiq.* **a** One who eats at the table of another, repaying him with flattery or buffoonery. **b** One of a class of assistants in religious rites who dined with the priests after a sacrifice.

2. One frequenting the tables of the rich, or living at another's expense, and earning his welcome by flattery; a hanger-on; a toady; a sycophant.

3. *Biol.* A plant or animal living in, on, or with some other living organism (called its *host*) at whose expense it is maintained (obtaining food, shelter, or some other advantage), but which usually it does not immediately destroy.

Webster's Third New International Dictionary[1]

No one likes to be called a parasite. It is a nasty word. However, its unpleasant connotations lie in the realm of human relations, not biological ones. From a non-anthropocentric viewpoint, parasitism is just one of the three great universal food-getting habits among non-photosynthetic organisms, the other two being the saprophytic and the predatory habits. The dictionary reveals that these words also have nasty derivations and meanings. This unsavory semantic situation results from a simple biological fact: all non-photosynthetic organisms[2] live by eating the bodies of other organisms. They are called "saprophytes," "predators," or

---

[1] By permission. Copyright 1961 by G. and C. Merriam Co., Publishers of the Merriam-Webster Dictionaries.

[2] The chemoautotrophic bacteria excepted.

"parasites" on the basis of their table manners at the common feast. Saprophytes feed upon organisms that are dead before they find them; predators eat organisms which they have killed themselves or had killed for them; and parasites consume their hosts piecemeal without bothering to kill them at all, at least not immediately.

This classification assumes the equality of all living things, as both diner and dinner, whether they are plants or animals, one-celled or many-celled. Thus a turkey buzzard feeding on a dead cow is as much a saprophyte as a bacterium decomposing a dead tree trunk, and a Jain sipping his vegetable broth through a gauze mask is just as much a predator as a tiger devouring a calf.

The trichotomy of saprophyte, predator, and parasite does not always adequately characterize food-getting habits, for there may exist almost every conceivable gradation between one habit and another within a group of closely related organisms living in a single environment. The enteric bacilli of the human bowel are almost indistinguishable on simple morphological grounds and share many common physiological and immunological properties. Yet they include, on the one hand, true saprophytes of soil, milk, plants, etc., which are only accidental inhabitants of the gut, and, on the other, true parasites, which cannot multiply outside the human body, and, in between the two clearly recognizable extremes, all the intermediate stages that anyone could wish for. More heterogeneous gradations between parasite and predator may also be recognized. The adult hookworm attaches itself to the intestinal wall and stays there indefinitely, feeding on its host's blood. The human head louse remains in intimate contact with its host but drinks his blood only intermittently. Other blood-feeders, such as leeches, horseflies, and mosquitos, live completely apart from their hosts except at mealtime, and, finally, some carnivores, after killing their prey, may drink only the blood and leave the carcass untouched.

Even the true parasitic habit itself is not a single way of life but a collection of many kinds of specific food-getting practices, all identified by the dependency of the parasite on the living host for its food. Since the hallmark of parasitism is a dependency on a living host for food, it should be possible to analyze the parasitic habit on the basis of the nature and degree of this dependency. Table I-1[3] is an attempt in this direction. Dependency is assessed in two ways: by the intimacy of association between host and parasite and by the food demands made upon the host by the parasite.

With respect to the first, four kinds of parasites may be recognized, and these are represented by the four vertical columns of Table I-1.

Facultative Parasites

Such organisms may live either as saprophytes or as parasites. A parasite may be considered capable of living a saprophytic life if it can exist for an indefinite number of generations without the intervention of any parasitic stage. Periods of parasitic existence are not obligatory, are probably accidental, and contribute little to the survival of the organism as a species. These casual parasites are indifferent dinner guests and cannot strictly be said to be dependent on their hosts at all.

Bacteria of the genus *Proteus* fit these requirements well. They are among the most common bacteria found in soil and in water and sewage laden with organic matter of animal origin. Their existence as saprophytes is unquestioned. Equally unquestioned is their role as pathogens. In man, they cause infections of the eye and ear, pleurisy,

[3] Table I-1 and all subsequent discussion are limited to consideration of single-celled parasites of animals.

TABLE I-1*

RELATION BETWEEN PARASITE HABIT AND NUTRITIONAL REQUIREMENT

PROBABLE NUTRITIONAL REQUIREMENTS DURING PARASITIC LIFE	Facultative Parasites	PARASITE HABIT			
		Obligate Parasites		Obligate Parasites	
		Obligate Extracellular	Facultative Intracellular	Obligate Intracellular	
Simple carbon and energy source, inorganic nitrogen	*Pseudomonas* *Escherichia*	Typhoid bacillus Cholera vibrio			
B vitamins, amino acids, nitrogen bases, etc.	*Clostridium* *Proteus*	*Staphylococcus* Dysentery bacillus Anthrax bacillus			
Complex natural materials—blood, serum, etc.		Trypanosomes *Streptococcus* *Pneumococcus* Diphtheria bacillus *Leptospira*	*Gonococcus* *Meningococcus* *Brucella* Tubercle bacillus	PPLO† *Bartonella*	
Unknown requirements satisfied only within living cells		Syphilis spirochete		Viruses Psittacosis group Rickettsiae Malarial parasites	

* Listing of specific organisms is for illustrative purposes only; it is not exhaustive. Classification is upon basis of most frequently encountered parasitic habit. Nutritional requirements often become simpler during continued cultivation in artificial media.

† Pleuropneumonia-like organisms.

peritonitis, wound infection, infant diarrhea, cystitis, and food poisoning. In addition to man, *Proteus* may infect other mammals, amphibia, and fishes.

The bacterial genus *Pseudomonas*, similarly found in water, soil, and all decaying organic matter, may nevertheless frequently parasitize and cause serious disease in insects, reptiles, birds, and mammals. In man himself, wound infections, middle-ear infections, endocarditis, pneumonia, dysentery, and generalized fatal septicemia may all be produced by pseudomonads.

Still another group of bacteria, the clostridia, have furnished several generations of bacteriology teachers with a near-perfect gradient between saprophyte and parasite. These bacteria are commonly found in the intestinal tract and in manured soils, but their isolation from virgin soils establishes their ability to live indefinitely as saprophytes. *Clostridium botulinum* is an obligate saprophyte with no power to invade and multiply in living tissues. It is responsible for the frequently fatal food poisoning known as "botulism" only because it elaborates a powerful toxin while growing in improperly preserved food. *C. tetani* produces a similar toxin in the tissues of its host to cause the symptoms of tetanus or lockjaw. However, it is unlikely that *C. tetani* can actually multiply in living tissues. Instead, it appears to grow only in tissues killed by the trauma of the wound itself or by the invasion of other bacteria. Finally, the organisms of gaseous gangrene, such as *C. welchii*, while dependent on trauma and other more invasive bacteria for their establishment in the body, can, once established, rapidly invade and multiply in healthy tissue.

In general, there are surprisingly few organisms that can be frank parasites or saprophytes as the occasion demands. It has always been tempting to see in such facultative parasites the evolutionary beginnings of parasitism, but it is by no means certain that this is true.

Obligate Parasites

In nature, these organisms multiply only within the bodies of their hosts. They may persist for a time in non-living natural environments, but they do not increase in number and would disappear as species in the absence of suitable hosts. This category includes the great bulk of single-celled parasites, and it is convenient to divide it into three subgroups, all fully dependent on intimate and more or less continuous association with their hosts and yet differing in the nature of this association:

A. *Obligate extracellular parasites*, multiplying only within the body cavities or the extracellular tissue spaces. Such parasites lack the ability to invade living cells actively and, when passively taken up by phagocytic cells, are destroyed or at least cease to multiply. As seen from Table I-1, the major fraction of the important pathogens of man are members of this group.

The factors which restrict an organism to an extracellular parasitic habitat are poorly understood. Many strict extracellular parasites would, from laboratory studies, appear to be perfectly capable of living in soil, water, and other natural habitats, and the special abilities required for successful intracellular growth are largely still unknown. Intracellular parasites are usually looked down on as weaklings lacking something required for life outside the cell, while it is seldom recognized that their more robust extracellular relatives lack something required for life inside the cell.

B. *Facultative intracellular parasites*, multiplying either extracellularly or within the cytoplasm or nucleus of host cells. The best-known members of this group are bacteria which cause in man extensive and severe diseases, such as gonorrhea, epidemic cerebrospinal meningitis, brucellosis undulant fever), tuberculosis, and tularemia. The cells in which they are found are almost invariably actively or potentially phagocytic cells, and it is not easy to decide whether the phagocyte or the bacterium is the victim. However, recent studies of experimental infections of phagocytes in tissue culture with tubercle bacilli and brucellae have clearly demonstrated the ability of these bacteria to multiply in and destroy phagocytes. The general failure to find organisms of this type within non-phagocytic cells suggests that they lack the ability to invade host cells actively but that, once taken up by phagocytes, they are able to multiply within an intracellular environment.

The role of intracellular multiplication in the survival of these organisms as species and in the pathology of the diseases they produce is not well defined. However, with respect to gonococci, brucellae, and tubercle bacilli, their ability to live within host cells may contribute to the prolonged infections characteristic of their diseases, a condition which would tend to favor wider dissemination of these agents and facilitate their survival.

Again, without substantial justification, this group of facultative organisms has frequently been considered the evolutionary forebear of the final group.

C. *Obligate intracellular parasites,* in nature multiplying only within other living cells. This is the special group of parasites with which this book will be concerned. Here the elective choice of the previous group is an absolute necessity. Both the survival of the species and the pathology of the disease are entirely dependent on intracellular multiplication. A glance at Table I-1 shows that no particular selectivity as to type of organism is achieved by this restriction. Protozoa, bacteria, and viruses may all be obligate intracellular parasites. Members of this group multiply in a much wider variety of host cell than do the facultative intracellular parasites; almost every kind of body cell may be

7

parasitized by one or more of these agents. Many of them have been demonstrated to invade cells with no phagocytic propinquities. Since we shall be concerned in later chapters with detailed consideration of several of these obligate intracellular parasites, let us proceed without further attention to the second way of estimating the degree and nature of the dependency of the parasite on the host for its food.

Ideally, the food demands of the parasite on the host should be determined by studying the nutritional requirements of the parasite as it grows in the tissues of an appropriate host. Unfortunately, however, present methods of nutritional investigation cannot handle such a complex situation. Therefore, it has been necessary to establish the growth requirements of parasites in artificial laboratory media and to extrapolate this information to the host-parasite relationship. With the exception of the obligate intracellular parasites, parasitic organisms can generally grow in non-living laboratory media, despite the fact that in nature many of them multiply only in association with their hosts. This immediately shows that food demand is not the sole determinant of parasitic habit; but let us see just what relationship between the two can be found.

For the parasites capable of multiplying in non-living media, the food requirements under these artificial conditions probably approximate their requirements in parasitic life. However, two important type of phenomena greatly lessen the value of this correlation. First, the food requirements of a parasite upon primary isolation from an infected host are frequently more complex than after many subcultures in artificial media. Staphylococci directly obtained from suppurative lesions usually require several amino acids, purines, nicotinic acid, thiamin, and biotin. Yet, upon continued cultivation, the growth medium can sometimes be progressively simplified until it contains only inorganic salts, glucose, and ammonia. Many other similar examples have long been known. Such alterations in food demand usually occur through the familiar process of mutation and selection, greatly encouraged by the enormous numbers of individuals present in each culture and by the short generation time of single-celled organisms. Spontaneous mutants with simpler growth needs grow faster and survive better in the artificial medium than the original major type in the primary isolate. Progressive simplification of the medium strongly favors the new types, the population equilibrium shifts in their favor, and the original type may be rapidly replaced by one with simplified growth needs and frequently with a much lower potential for parasitic life. For this reason, only the behavior of a parasite immediately after recovery from an infected host is of any real value in estimating its nutritional status in parasitic life.

The second phenomenon involves, not mutation and selection, but the immediate response of the entire parasite population to its environment. An organism perfectly capable of synthesizing the purine adenine may, when supplied with the purine in its growth medium, cease to synthesize adenine and use the adenine of the medium to make its nucleic acids. Thus the failure of an organism to exhibit a need for a particular substance, even on primary isolation, does not necessarily mean that the host does not supply it to the parasite. The evolutionist, speculating on the origin of parasitism, finds here a fascinating clue.

Returning to Table I-1, the food demands of the parasite on the host are arranged in the four horizontal columns, opposing the four types of host-parasite association just discussed. For the reasons given, the growth requirements indicated are those generally observed on primary isolation and are best regarded as an approximation of the minimum demands of the parasite upon its host.

Parasites Requiring Only a Simple Carbon Source and Inorganic Nitrogen

These organisms have all the enzymic machinery required to obtain from a simple organic compound such as glucose the carbon skeletons of all its organic constituents, as well as the energy necessary for such syntheses. Organic nitrogen compounds are obtained by incorporating the nitrogen of ammonia into the carbon skeletons provided by the simple carbon source. Thus they require no specific organic compounds, merely carbon in organic form as raw material and as a source of energy.

Organisms with so simple a nutritional requirement are rarely capable of leading a true parasitic existence, although there is no clear reason why this should be so. Conversely, there is no simple explanation of why the typhoid bacillus, which can grow on glucose and ammonia, fails to multiply in nature outside its human host.

Parasites Requiring One or More Specific Organic Nitrogen Compounds

These parasites can also convert simple carbon compounds and ammonia to complex cell material, but, because of synthetic deficiencies, they cannot make all their cell constituents in this manner and must receive some of them in their diet. For example, *Proteus* will grow on glucose and ammonia if supplied with a single B vitamin—nicotinic acid. Other parasites of this group may require a number of specific growth substances. The requirements of freshly isolated staphylococci just described furnish a typical example.

Parasites Requiring Complex Natural Materials

On fresh isolation from infected hosts, such organisms do not grow, or grow only sparsely, in media of known chemical composition. They are usually cultured in media enriched with complex natural materials, such as blood, serum, or ascitic fluid. They must receive from their hosts growth substances of as yet unknown composition. The substances may conceivably be polymers of known substances, such as polypeptides and polynucleotides, or they may be compounds of an as yet unrecognized nature.

This group contains parasites with widely varying parasitic habits. There are obviously no facultative parasites with such growth requirements, but, not so obviously, some forms which in their hosts behave as obligate intracellular parasites may multiply in the test tube in appropriate complex media (Table I-1).

Parasites Growing Only in the Presence of Living Cells

These organisms demand something from their hosts that only living cells can provide. Most of them are obligate intracellular parasites, the only important exceptions being the spirochetes of syphilis and relapsing fever. They include the small true viruses (which are probably not true organisms in the sense of this discussion), the micro-organisms of the psittacosis group, the rickettsiae, the leprosy bacillus, and the vertebrate-inhabiting forms of protozoa, such as malarial parasites and the agents of kala-azar.

With Table I-1 completed, we see that there is a good correlation between the intimacy of association between host and parasite and the food demands—the nutritional requirements—of the parasite. The correlation is not perfect, for parasitism is a complex phenomenon and yields to no single explanation. However, obligate intracellular parasitism emerges as an extreme example of the metabolic dependency of the parasite on the host. In succeeding chapters, several intracellular parasite-host systems will be examined in detail, and it will be seen that, even at this extreme, there is a wide variation in the relative magnitude of the metabolic

11

contribution of host and parasite toward the reproduction of the parasite.

Two main kinds of obligate intracellular parasites may be recognized: the organismal type and the viral type. Organismal parasites are clearly micro-organisms. They satisfy the conventional definitions of organism, reproduce by division of existing units, and have obviously evolved from ancestors capable of living by themselves. Viruses do not at all satisfy usual definitions of organisms, and their origin is a matter of energetic and generally fruitless speculation. They reproduce by separate synthesis of relatively simple subunits and subsequent assembly into new complete ones. The viral type of obligate intracellular parasitism has been thoroughly discussed in recent books ranging from the small volume of Weidel (1959) to the encyclopedic treatise edited by Burnet and Stanley (1959). We shall concern ourselves here with the relatively neglected organismal type and with the pox viruses, which in some respects bridge the gap between the two great groups.

The unique problem in the multiplication of obligate intracellular parasites of both types is not how they reproduce themselves. Their chemical composition and enzymic machinery (when there is any present) are closely similar to the host cells in which they grow, and we can be sure that the same general types of enzyme systems are responsible for the synthesis of both host and parasite protoplasm. The real problem is why the intracellular parasites grow so well within suitable host cells and so poorly outside them.

REFERENCES

BURNET, F. M., and STANLEY, W. M. 1959. The viruses. 3 vols. New York: Academic Press.

WEIDEL, W. 1959. Virus. Ann Arbor: University of Michigan Press.

CHAPTER II

The Malarial Parasites

Malarial parasites are the largest and most complex of the obligate intracellular parasites that we shall consider. It is not surprising, then, that for these organisms we can define most precisely the metabolic role of both parasite and host in parasite reproduction and come closest to locating the biochemical lesions that restrict them to an intracellular existence. Malarial parasites are Protozoa belonging to a single genus *Plasmodium*. They are the most important members of the relatively small class Sporozoa, a group of uncertain relationship to the other Protozoa. Different species of *Plasmodium* cause malaria in man, other mammals, birds, and reptiles. Man himself is the host for four different species of plasmodia, and, despite tremendous advances in the control of malaria, it still remains the commonest and the costliest infectious disease of man.

In order to survive as a species in nature, the malarial parasite must live alternately in vertebrate and invertebrate hosts. In their vertebrate hosts, the parasites multiply asexually in the red blood cells. A small fraction of the asexual blood forms differentiate into sexual stages which develop no further unless ingested by a suitable mosquito host, whereupon fertilization occurs in the insect's stomach, and the zygotes invade the cells of the stomach wall and begin to multiply. Eventually, infective forms known as "sporozoites" are formed and accumulate in the salivary glands, from which they are injected into a new vertebrate host while the mosquito is feeding. The sporozoites do not, as once thought, directly invade the erythrocytes of the new host. Instead, they go through several cycles of asexual reproduction in the macrophages of the skin and the endothelial cells lining the blood vessels before forms capable of invading red blood cells appear and complete the life-cycle.

Much could certainly be learned by studying the metabolic interaction of plasmodium and host cell at each stage of the life-cycle, for the differential susceptibility to drugs exhibited by the same species of parasite growing in the mosquito, in non-erythrocytic cells of the vertebrate host, and in its erythrocytes strongly hints that metabolic shifts accompany the various steps in the life-cycle. Unfortunately, even with modern micromethods, relatively huge numbers of parasites are required for metabolic studies, and these are available only in the blood stages. In fact, only the most severe animal malarias in which almost every red blood cell becomes infected furnish enough parasites to satisfy the biochemist. For these reasons, metabolic studies have been largely restricted to the blood forms of three species: *P. knowlesi* in the monkey, *P. gallinaceum* in the chicken, and *P. lophurae* in the duck. Cultivation experiments in which the plasmodia are allowed to multiply in vitro within suitable host cells require much fewer parasites, and all stages in the life-cycle have been studied in this manner. Here again extensive studies on the in vitro nutritional requirements of malarial parasites have been carried out only with the blood stages of *P. knowlesi* and *P. lophurae*. However, what little we do know about other species, including the human ones, suggests that there are no major biochemical differences among the various members of the genus *Plasmodium*.

GROWTH, MORPHOLOGY, AND CHEMICAL COMPOSITION
OF THE BLOOD STAGES

Biochemical studies on intracellular host-parasite systems are most valuable when they can be correlated with the morphological development of the parasite and the concomitant morphological alterations in the host. Because of the experimental restrictions just described, we need be concerned here only with the asexual cycle in the red blood cells. The earliest stage is about one-fifth the diameter of its host cell. It grows rapidly, and soon the nucleus begins to divide. Growth and nuclear division continue until the parasite nearly fills the red cell and 16–32 nuclei are present. Then the cytoplasm about each nucleus separates, and a new daughter cell is formed; the host cell disintegrates, the daughter cells are released into the blood, and a large proportion of them find their way into new erythrocytes to complete the asexual cycle. This cycle takes 24 hours in *P. knowlesi* and 36 hours in *P. gallinaceum* and *P. lophurae*. If we assume the production of 16 new daughter cells in 24 hours, this would give a doubling time of 6 hours. While this is less than that of a fast-growing bacterium in a good medium, which may show a doubling time of half an hour, it is indicative of a respectable rate of multiplication and synthesis of new cell material.

Recent electron-microscopic observations on thin sections of parasitized erythrocytes have shown that the fine structure of the malarial parasite is very similar to that of other cells (Fulton and Flewett, 1956; Rudzinska and Trager, 1957, 1959). Figure II-1 shows a thin section of a rat erythrocyte containing a young form of *P. berghei*. The parasite is clearly visible because its cytoplasm is much less electron-dense than that of its host. The parasite is surrounded by a double cytoplasmic membrane in close contact with host cytoplasm. Its own cytoplasm contains little endoplasmic reticulum and few

15

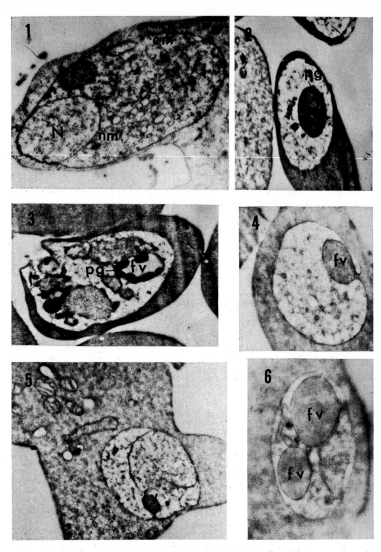

Figs. II-1–II-6.—Electron micrographs of thin sections of osmium-fixed erythrocytes infected with malarial parasites. Figs. II-1, -4, -5, and -6 are from Rudzinska and Trager (1959) and are reproduced by permission of the authors and the *Journal of Biophysical and Biochemical Cytology.* Figs. III-2 and -3 are from Rudzinska and Trager (1957) and are reproduced by permission of the authors and the *Journal of Protozoology.*

Fig. II-1: Rat erythrocyte infected with a young form of *P. berghei.* 14,000×. N = nucleus, nm = nuclear membrane, cm = cytoplasmic membrane, fv = food vacuole. Fig. II-2: *P. lophurae* in a duck erythrocyte. Section through a young parasite showing a large food vacuole with pigment granules (pg) inside. 8,000×. Fig. II-3: Like Fig. 2. Section through a late-stage parasite. 8,000×. Fig. II-4: *P. berghei* in a rat erythrocyte. The food vacuole is still connected with the cytoplasm of the host. 14,000×. Fig. II-5: Like Fig. 4. The food vacuole is connected with the host cytoplasm by a narrow neck. 14,000×. Fig. II-6: Like Fig. 4. Two food vacuoles are present. One is in the last stages of pinching off, and the process has been completed in the other. 20,000×.

mitochondria. The nucleus is surrounded by a double nuclear membrane. In general, the fine structure of malarial parasites appears relatively simple.

The chemical composition of malarial parasites has been deduced by comparing parasitized with non-parasitized erythrocytes and directly determined by analyzing free parasites released from their host cells by a hemolytic agent. Neither method yields results of high precision and reliability, but they both show clearly that the chemical composition of plasmodia is as complex as that of their host cells. The parasites have an unusually high content of lipids, but this is about their only analytical oddity.

Metabolic Pathways

Biochemical research on the malarial parasites has been concentrated in two areas—metabolic pathways and nutritional requirements. Each kind of study has repeatedly aided and complemented the other, and neither can really be discussed independently. However, it is convenient and, we hope, less confusing to discuss, first, the metabolic mechanisms and then the nutritional needs of plasmodia.

Carbohydrate Metabolism

Suspensions of parasitized erythrocytes maintained in vitro support growth and multiplication of the plasmodia only when glucose or a few other related sugars are present. Comparatively little glucose is assimilated into new parasite protoplasm; most of it is oxidized to furnish energy for biosynthetic purposes.

Glucose disappears very rapidly from parasitized erythrocyte suspensions, some twenty-five to one hundred times as fast as from uninfected ones. In the absence of oxygen, all the utilized glucose is converted to lactate, but in the presence of oxygen, a quarter to a half of it is oxidized completely to car-

17

bon dioxide and water (Wendel, 1943; Silverman *et al.*, 1944; McKee *et al.*, 1946). The mechanism of glucose breakdown has been worked out in detail for *P. gallinaceum*, and enough is known about glucose degradation in other species for us to be reasonably certain that results with this species apply generally.

Further studies on mechanisms of carbohydrate metabolism had to be carried out with plasmodia freed from their erythrocyte hosts. Most of the intermediates in glucose metabolism are highly polar substances, such as phosphorylated sugars and polycarboxylic acids, which penetrate the cell membrane of the erythrocyte very slowly, if at all, and are thus not available to the parasite within.

The quantitative anaerobic conversion of glucose to lactate makes it look very much as if malarial parasites degrade glucose by way of a phosphorylating glycolysis or Embden-Meyerhof cycle. In general, the enzymes of this cycle are all soluble and readily extracted from cells. Therefore, Speck and Evans (1945) used cell-free extracts in their study of the initial attack on glucose by plasmodia. They lysed chicken erythrocytes parasitized with *P. gallinaceum* with the hemolytic glycoside saponin and ground the freed parasites with powdered glass. The extracts obtained in this way carried out three key reactions of the Embden-Meyerhof cycle: the phosphorylation of glucose by ATP,[1] the cleavage of fructose-1,6-diphosphate to 3-phosphoglyceraldehyde, and the coupled oxidation-reduction reaction between 3-phosphoglyceraldehyde and pyruvate (see Diagram II-1).

Since parasitized erythrocytes oxidize pyruvate at the same rate as glucose or lactate, it seems likely that the plasmodia, like many other organisms, form pyruvate by glycoly-

[1] The following abbreviations will be used: DNA = Deoxyribonucleic acid. RNA = Ribonucleic acid. DPN = Diphosphopyridine nucleotide. TPN = Triphosphopyridine nucleotide. ATP = Adenosine triphosphate. ADP = Adenosine diphosphate. Co A = Coenzyme A. *p*AB = *p*-Aminobenzoic acid.

sis and then oxidize it completely via the Krebs tricarboxylic acid cycle (Diagram II-2). The enzymes of this cycle are not readily brought into solution, and Speck, Moulder, and Evans (1946) studied the mechanism of pyruvate oxidation in intact free parasites of *P. gallinaceum*. Parasites liberated by saponin had weak and erratic oxidative powers, and success was achieved only when free parasites were produced by

DIAGRAM II-1

The Embden-Meyerhof Glycolytic Cycle

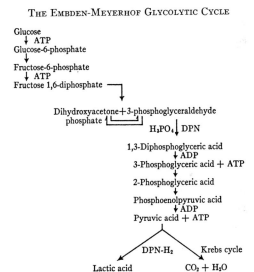

the lysis of infected red cells with guinea-pig complement and anti-erythrocyte hemolytic antibody produced in rabbits by immunization with normal chicken red cells.

In his studies on pyruvate oxidation in muscle, Krebs set up several conditions that had to be met in order that it might be concluded that a tricarboxylic acid cycle was operating in a given cell or tissue. All these were met for pyruvate oxidation in free parasites of *P. gallinaceum*. They are, briefly,

19

(1) the acids of the cycle were oxidized as fast as pyruvate itself; (2) the oxidation of pyruvate was catalyzed by small amounts of the dicarboxylic acids of the Krebs cycle; (3) traces of citrate accumulated during pyruvate oxidation; and (4) pyruvate oxidation was strongly inhibited by malonate, a specific inhibitor of succinate oxidation, and succinate accumulated during the oxidation of pyruvate in the presence of fumarate and malonate. The significance of these observations will be apparent from examination of Diagram II-2.

DIAGRAM II-2

THE KREBS TRICARBOXYLIC ACID CYCLE

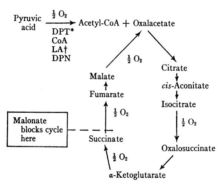

* DPT = diphosphothiamin.   † LA = α-Lipoic acid.

The energy liberated from glucose during glycolysis to lactate and during complete oxidation to carbon dioxide and water appears to be conserved and utilized for metabolic purposes in the form of the high-energy phosphate bonds of ATP, just as in other organisms whose energy metabolism is better understood. In the glycolytic cycle, Speck and Evans (1945) gave good indirect evidence for believing that ATP was formed from inorganic phosphate and ADP during the oxidation of 3-phosphoglyceraldehyde in extracts of *P. gallinaceum* (Diagram II-1). Bovarnick, Lindsay, and Hellerman (1946) showed that the oxidation of glucose by free parasites of *P. lophurae* was accompanied by the uptake of inorganic phosphate into organic linkage and that this uptake was accelerated by the addition of acids of the Krebs cycle.

Most of the metabolically available energy of glucose is not liberated in glycolysis but is still present in the pyruvate molecule when it enters the Krebs cycle, and consequently almost ten times as much ATP is formed during the complete oxidation of one molecule of glucose via the Krebs cycle as from its glycolysis to two molecules of lactate. However, plasmodia convert four to six molecules of glucose to lactate for every one they oxidize completely. Thus roughly comparable yields of energy are obtained from glycolysis and the tricarboxylic acid cycle. The success of Anfinsen *et al.* (1946) in cultivating *P. knowlesi* in parasitized monkey erythrocytes maintained under very low oxygen tensions has shown that, when necessary, the malarial parasite can obtain all its energy from glycolysis. Clarke (1952*b*) later obtained similar results with *P. gallinaceum* growing in chicken erythrocytes in vitro.

We may safely conclude from all these studies that the malarial parasite possesses the same mechanisms for the breakdown of glucose as does its vertebrate host and that we must look elsewhere for an explanation of its obligate intracellular parasitism. However, there are some very suggestive differences between the metabolic behavior of parasitized erythrocytes and free parasites to which we shall return at the end of this chapter.

Protein Metabolism

Plasmodial blood stages must synthesize protein at a rate commensurate with their rapid increase in size and number. Since free-living protozoans, whose nutritional requirements are known, have only limited abilities to make amino acids from ammonia and appropriate carbon sources, we may assume that parasite protein is made almost entirely from pre-formed amino acids of the host. The contribution of the free amino acids present in the erythrocyte at time of infection may be dismissed as being too small to be significant, leaving, as possible sources of plasmodial protein, the free amino acids of the serum, the serum proteins, and the proteins of the host red cell. The free amino acids of the serum would seem to be a logical source of building material for parasite protein, but the nutritional studies of McKee and Geiman (1948) and the isotopic labeling investigations of Fulton and Grant (1956) have shown that, except for a single amino acid—methionine —the uptake of the free serum amino acids into parasite protein is not required for their growth and multiplication. The serum proteins contain large amounts of methionine, but the parasites cannot use it. Thus, by elimination, we are left with the protein of the erythrocyte as the chief source of parasite protein. About 90 per cent of the red cell protein is hemoglobin; so, to be more specific, the chief source of para-site protein must be hemoglobin. There is abundant evidence that the malarial parasites actively metabolize hemoglobin, and most studies on the protein metabolism of plasmodia have concentrated on the breakdown and utilization of hemo-globin by the parasites.

The breakdown of hemoglobin is made visibly evident by the formation of parasite pigment, which was, in fact, dis-covered before the parasites themselves. Early pathologists recognized the connection between malaria and pigmented bodies in the liver and spleen long before Laveran discovered the parasites in the red blood cells. As the plasmodium grows inside the red cell, minute granules of a dense, highly re-fractile pigment appear in its cytoplasm. These granules in-crease in number, clump together, and are released into the serum when the red cell disintegrates at the close of the asex-ual cycle. It was assumed very early that the malarial pigment was formed by the breakdown of hemoglobin. In 1911, Brown foreshadowed present ideas by postulating that malarial parasites contained an enzyme that cleaves hemoglobin into its protein component globin and the iron porphyrin hematin. He believed that the globin was utilized in the growth of the parasite but that hematin was merely a waste product. Proof of his hypotheses had to await the discovery of suitable experimental malarias, such as *P. knowlesi* and *P. gallinaceum*, and the development of adequate methods for preparing parasites essentially free of host material and for studying the changes in the various nitrogenous fractions of the host cell during the growth of the parasite.

A large number of investigations, beginning with the pioneering efforts of Sinton and Ghosh (1934) and culminating with the modern analytical work of Deegan and Maegraith (1956), have established beyond any doubt that the pigment produced by a number of animal and human malarias is hematin. The results of Deegan and Maegraith strongly indicate that it is not free hematin but this compound combined with denatured protein or polypeptide. Deegan and Maegraith have pointed out that hematin is a potent inhibitor of succinic dehydrogenase (Keilin and Hartree, 1947), which we have seen to be a key enzyme in the oxidation of glucose by plasmodia, while hematin coupled with another nitrogenous compound is not. It is not known whether such coupling occurs before or after the cleavage of hemoglobin.

Brown's hypothesis that the first step in the metabolism of hemoglobin by malarial parasites is its cleavage into hematin and globin has been indirectly verified for *P. knowlesi* and *P. gallinaceum* by several different groups (Sinton and Ghosh, 1934; Christophers and Fulton, 1938; Ball *et al.*, 1948; Morrison and Jeskey, 1948; Groman, 1951). They all showed that, as the parasite grows in the erythrocyte, there is a drastic reduction in the hemoglobin content and a corresponding rise in malarial pigment. In infections with *P. knowlesi*, as much as three-fourths of the hemoglobin may be destroyed during the 24 hours that the plasmodium is growing in the erythrocyte. In *P. gallinaceum*-infected red cells, the corresponding maximum destruction is somewhat less.

An isolated plasmodial enzyme system capable of cleaving hemoglobin into hematin and globin is still to be demonstrated. This is disappointing, because such a reaction appears to be unique to the malarial parasites, the normal vertebrate pathway of hemoglobin breakdown being via the bile pigments. This perhaps explains why the malarial pigment remains so long in the macrophages, which ingest it after disintegration of the infected red cell.

Brown's prediction that the globin part of hemoglobin is further utilized by the parasite has also found experimental support. Erythrocytes parasitized with *P. knowlesi* or *P. gallinaceum* form such large quantities of free amino acids that they can have come from no other source than the hemoglobin (Moulder and Evans, 1946; Morrison and Jeskey, 1948; Groman, 1951). In addition, extracts of *P. gallinaceum*, *P. knowlesi*, and *P. berghei* hydrolyze globin and denatured hemoglobin with the liberation of free amino acids (Moulder and Evans, 1946; Cook *et al.*, 1961). The latter workers have shown that this proteolytic activity is due to parasite enzymes and not to those of the red cell hosts. The accumulation of free amino acids indicates that the potentiality for the hydrolysis of host protein is greater than that for the incorporation of the resulting amino acids into parasite protein.

Such incorporation was strongly suggested from the balance studies of Morrison and Jeskey (1948). Fulton and Grant (1956) completed the proof when they showed that when the hemoglobin of monkey erythrocytes was labeled in vivo with the radioisotope of sulfur, S^{35}, the sulfur amino acids methionine and cystine were rapidly incorporated into the protein of *P. knowlesi* growing inside the labeled red cells.

Since it seemed unlikely that intact hemoglobin molecules could pass freely through the limiting membranes of parasites into their cytoplasm, it was assumed without direct evidence that plasmodia secrete extracellular enzymes which break down hemoglobin into hematin and amino acids. It could be further assumed that the amino acids were taken up by the parasites for protein synthesis; but this left the malarial pigment embarrassingly situated in the host cytoplasm instead of in the parasite cytoplasm, where it should have been. A much more satisfying picture of the gross aspects of hemoglobin digestion has been given by the electron-microscopic studies of Rudzinska and Trager (1957, 1959) on *P. lophurae* and *P. berghei*. Their thin-section electron micrographs show that the parasites feed by phagotrophy; that is, they engulf portions of the red cell cytoplasm by invaginating their limiting membranes. Figures II-4, II-5, and II-6 show successive stages in this process. The accumulation of pigment granules in the food vacuoles leaves little doubt that they are the site of hemoglobin digestion (Figs. II-2 and II-3). The completed vacuole is entirely incased in a membrane that was once a part of the original limiting membrane of the parasite; hence we must still postulate the secretion of hemoglobin-splitting enzymes—but secretion into the food vacuole and not into the host cytoplasm.

These morphologic observations furnish a plausible explanation for the curious linking of hemoglobin breakdown with aerobic oxidative processes (Moulder and Evans, 1946; Groman, 1951). When the aerobic oxidation of glucose is interfered with, as by removal of oxygen or by addition of inhibitors such as cyanide or malonate, there is a decrease in the accumulation of free amino acids, although protein hydrolysis is not an energy-requiring process. It now seems likely that the oxidative energy is needed for the formation of the food vacuole and for the secretion of the hemoglobin-digesting enzymes into it.

The finding that malarial parasites take up hemoglobin by phagotrophy may also explain the relation between sickle-cell anemia and resistance to malaria (see Lehmann, 1959). Allison (1954) found that the gene which produced sickle-cell anemia in its homozygous condition made its heterozygous carriers more resistant to *P. falciparum* (malignant tertian malaria) in their infancy. From the work of Pauling and his associates (1949), we know that the sickling gene causes the synthesis of an abnormal hemoglobin—hemoglobin S—instead of the normal hemoglobin A. Red blood cells of homozygous individuals contain only hemoglobin S, while those of heterozygotic individuals contain both hemoglobin S and hemoglobin A. Ingram (1959) has demonstrated that the two hemoglobins differ only in a single amino acid in each of the two identical halves of the hemoglobin molecule. In hemoglobin S, a neutral valine residue has been substituted for an acidic glutamic acid residue. This reduction in charge lessens the solubility of the reduced hemoglobin S to only about one-fiftieth that of the normal molecule, and solutions containing only a few per cent hemoglobin S become very viscous. From the extensive information on the specificity of such proteinases as pepsin and trypsin, it seems unlikely that a change in a single amino acid residue would make the hemoglobin molecule resistant to the plasmodial proteinases. However, the great increase in the viscosity of the cytoplasm of host red cells containing hemoglobin S could easily interfere with the phagotrophy of host material by the parasites and thus make individuals with hemoglobin S in their red cells more resistant to malaria.

As already indicated, the only plasmodial amino acid requirement not satisfied by hemoglobin is the one for the sulfur-containing amino acid methionine. When McKee *et al.* (1947) made this discovery, they thought that perhaps the methionine in the red cell hemoglobin was insufficient to meet the needs of the growing parasite, but Fulton and Grant (1956) have more recently shown that the situation is more complex. They measured the amount of methionine in monkey erythrocytes and in isolated parasites of *P. knowlesi* and found that the erythrocyte hemoglobin contains more than six times as much methionine as is needed for synthesis of parasite protein.

However, in confirmation of McKee *et al.* (1947), they reported that, during in vivo growth of *P. knowlesi* in S^{35}-labeled erythrocytes, only 80 per cent of the methionine of the parasite protein came from the hemoglobin of the host erythrocyte. According to the arguments already presented, the other 20 per cent must come from the serum, a conclusion confirmed by Fulton and Grant's demonstration of the rapid incorporation of free extracellular S^{35}-methionine into *P. knowlesi* during artificial cultivation. They also demonstrated that an appreciable amount of the cystine of parasite protein was derived from methionine. Thus it appears that the rate of liberation of methionine from hemoglobin is not sufficient to meet the needs for direct incorporation into parasite protein and conversion into cystine and that an extracellular supply of the amino acid is required for maximum parasite growth.

It should then be expected that the supply of free methionine may be the rate-limiting factor for parasite growth. That this is actually true is shown by the demonstration by McKee and Geiman (1948) that the inhibition of *P. knowlesi* multiplication produced by fasting the host may be relieved by feeding methionine and that parasite growth is inhibited by a methionine analogue—methoxinine—and the inhibition in turn relieved by methionine itself.

Nucleic Acid Metabolism

All the available studies suggest that the nucleic acid metabolism of plasmodia is similar to that of other organisms. They have a nucleus containing DNA and a cytoplasm rich in RNA (Lewert, 1952a). Mammalian erythrocytes contain little or no DNA, while the nucleated avian red cells contain large amounts. Both have low concentrations of RNA. Ball *et al.* (1948) demonstrated that monkey erythrocytes parasitized with *P. knowlesi* showed large increases in total nucleic acid during the growth of the parasites in vitro and in vivo. Whitfield (1953a) found much larger amounts of RNA and DNA in rat reticulocytes parasitized with *P. berghei* than in unparasitized ones. These increases must have come from the *de novo* synthesis of nucleic acid from non-erythrocytic precursors, as is indicated by the rapid uptake of radioactive phosphorus in plasmodial RNA and DNA during growth (Clarke, 1952a; Whitfield, 1953b). Lewert (1952b) studied the synthesis of both kinds of nucleic acid by *P. gallinaceum* growing in chicken red cells in vivo and concluded that the breakdown of the nuclear DNA of the host cell contributed heavily to the synthesis of new parasite nucleic acid.

Lipid Metabolism

The few investigations of the lipids of the malarial parasite have all been confined to *P. knowlesi*. There are large increases in the lipid content of parasitized monkey erythrocytes during the growth of the parasites in vitro and in vivo (Ball *et al.*, 1948; Morrison and Jeskey, 1948). This is because the parasites themselves have a very high lipid content, almost 30 per cent of the dry weight according to Morrison and Jeskey (1947). Neutral fat, phospholipid, and cholesterol are all present.

Nutritional Requirements

Attempts at obtaining growth and multiplication of malarial parasites outside their vertebrate hosts were generally unsuccessful until after the explosive advances in microbial metabolism and nutrition in the late 1930's and early 1940's and the application of this new knowledge to the study of plasmodial metabolism.

Requirements for Growth of Malarial Parasites within Erythrocytes Maintained in Vitro

Most of the work has been done by Trager with *P. lophurae* in duck red cells and by Ball, Geiman, McKee, Anfinson, and their associates with *P. knowlesi* in monkey cells. The latter workers also made limited studies on a number of other malarial parasites, and it seems reasonably safe to assume that the major nutritional needs of all species of plasmodia are the same under these conditions.

In a red cell–parasite system, two main kinds of cultural requirements will be evident—those of the red cell and those of the parasite. While maintenance of the erythrocyte in good condition is absolutely essential for the successful cultivation of intracellular plasmodia, it is the second type of nutritional requirement in which we are most interested here, and the first set of cultural needs will be dismissed by noting that such factors as tonicity and ionic composition of the suspending medium, pH, oxygen tension, and carbon dioxide tension must be carefully regulated. The glucose rapidly utilized by the growing parasites must be replaced, and the lactate and other plasmodial metabolic end-products must be removed. When these requirements are met, successful satisfaction of the special needs of the parasites allows in vitro growth and multiplication of the plasmodia equal to that obtained in the blood stream of an intact infected animal.

29

In his early studies on the cultivation of *P. lophurae* in duck red cells, Trager (1941, 1943) found that glutathione and pantothenate favored the growth and multiplication of the parasites. While both these substances, pantothenate in particular, are probably specific parasite requirements, it remained for Anfinsen *et al.* (1946) to find the first unequivocal parasite need. They had already obtained multiplication of *P. knowlesi* in monkey red cells suspended in a medium containing, among numerous ingredients, proteose-peptone, a familiar component of bacterial culture media. They were able to replace this complex protein digest with a few micrograms of *p*AB, one of the precursors of the B vitamin folic acid, which, in its coenzyme form, is a cofactor for many important biosynthetic reactions in which various one-carbon units are transferred from one molecule to another. The significance of this finding lies in the fact that higher animals cannot make folic acid from *p*AB but must have the complete vitamin supplied in their diets. Thus the *p*AB requirement of the red cell–parasite system must be referred to the parasite partner. The inhibition of plasmodial multiplication in vivo by sulfonamides, which are known to interfere with the formation of folic acid from *p*AB, and the reversal of the sulfonamide inhibition by *p*AB itself are further evidence for this conclusion (see Rollo, 1955). All these observations suggest that malarial parasites synthesize folic acid from *p*AB and other simple substances.

The other specific parasite requirement definitely demonstrated in the red blood cell–parasite in vitro system is methionine. Anfinsen *et al.* (1946) were able to replace the plasma of their original suspending medium with bovine serum albumin. With this advance, they then established that multiplication of *P. knowlesi* was greatly increased by the addition of free amino acids in the form of a casein hydrolyzate (McKee *et al.*, 1947). McKee and Geiman (1948) next showed that the effect of the hydrolyzate could be duplicated by a single amino acid, L-methionine.

It is very interesting that the growth-stimulating action of either methionine or *p*AB is enhanced by the addition of the other. We know that methionine is synthesized by the addition of a one-carbon unit to homocysteine, a form of folic acid acting as cofactor. Once formed, it acts as a donor of methyl groups; again a folic acid cofactor is involved. However, the exact nature of the metabolic relationship between methionine and *p*AB in malarial parasites is still not known.

Although other requirements have not been clearly defined, they certainly exist. Addition of a whole array of B vitamins or all the commonly occurring purines or pyrimidines to the serum albumin–methionine-*p*AB-pantothenate system increases the intra-erythrocytic growth rate of *P. knowlesi* (Anfinsen *et al.*, 1946) and *P. lophurae* (Trager, 1947). It is disappointing that repeated attempts to obtain positive results with single members of these groups have all failed. Dialyzable extracts of liver and plasma will also increase the growth rate of *P. knowlesi* in red cells suspended in the serum albumin–methionine-*p*AB medium. Therefore, it is evident that there are as yet unidentified low-molecular-weight growth factors for plasmodia, but it is not clear whether they are merely the proper combination of known factors or new ones unique to the malarial parasite.

Requirements for the Survival and Development of Malarial Parasites outside the Erythrocyte

Most of the ambiguities inherent in studying the nutritional requirements of the red cell–parasite complex would disappear if plasmodia could be induced to grow and multiply outside their host cells. Trager has gone a long way toward reaching this goal in his attempts at the extracellular cultivation of *P. lophurae*. While he did not achieve significant ne multiplication, his parasites survived in good condition outside the red cell for as long as 3 days and developed from the small, mononucleated form to the large, multinucleated stages.

The basic medium for extracellular cultivation consisted essentially of the medium developed for growing the parasites inside red cells plus a concentrated extract of duck red cells and 6 per cent gelatin. Duck erythrocytes parasitized with the mononucleated stages of *P. lophurae* were suspended in this medium and hemolyzed with rabbit antiserum and guinea-pig complement. The resulting free parasites were then used as inoculum for the culture flasks, which were aerated at 40° C.

The basal medium gave good extracellular survival of *P. lophurae* for only about 1 day, but the successive addition of a number of well-known metabolites progressively lengthened the period of survival and development. The first such substances discovered were ATP, DPN, and pyruvate (Trager, 1950). Their addition gave almost 100 per cent survival for 2 days. The further addition of malate allowed some parasites to survive in good condition through the third day of extracellular life (Clarke, 1952*b;* Trager, 1952, 1954).

Although pantothenate was effective in promoting plasmodial growth in the red cell, it had no effect on extraerythrocytic survival. However, its coenzyme form—Co A—in conjunction with the other survival-promoting factors just listed allowed almost all the parasites to survive for 3 days in excellent condition (Trager, 1952). The difference in activity between pantothenate and Co A suggests that the free parasite cannot make the coenzyme, a possibility to be considered in the next section.

A possibly analogous situation exists with *p*AB and leucovorin (N_5-formyl-tetrahydrofolic acid). *p*AB is an active growth factor in parasitized erythrocytes (Anfinsen *et al.,*

1946), but only leucovorin prolongs extracellular survival (Trager, 1958). However, interpretation is difficult here because the conversion of pAB into forms of folic acid is not supposed to occur in vertebrate cells (see next section).

There is some evidence (Trager, 1958) that the red cell extracts furnish not only hemoglobin as the main nitrogen source but also other high-molecular-weight substances,

TABLE II-1

COMPARISON OF EXTRACELLULAR REQUIREMENTS FOR SURVIVAL AND FOR PYRUVATE OXIDATION IN MALARIAL PARASITES

Requirements for Extracellular Survival of *P. lophurae* (Trager, 1950, 1952, 1954, 1958)	Requirements for Extracellular Oxidation of Pyruvate by *P. gallinaceum* (Speck *et al.*, 1946)
Pyruvate	
Diphosphopyridine nucleotide	Di- and triphosphopyridine nucleotide
Adenosine triphosphate	Adenosine triphosphate
Malate	Malate (or other C_4 dicarboxylic acid)
Coenzyme A	
Leucovorin	
Red cell extract	Diphosphothiamin
Gelatin	Manganous chloride

which function as growth factors. Clarke (1952*b*) has also shown that the red cell lysate is essential for the survival of extracellular forms of *P. gallinaceum*.

The substances shown to favor the extracellular survival and development of *P. lophurae* are summarized in Table II-1.

SOME SPECULATIONS ON THE NATURE OF THE RESTRICTION OF THE MALARIAL PARASITE TO AN INTRACELLULAR EXISTENCE

Inside its host erythrocyte, the malarial parasite synthesizes new parasite material at such a rate that 16–32 new daughter cells are produced every 24–36 hours. Most of the materials necessary for this rapid growth are present within the erythrocyte, the only well-defined substances which must be taken into the red cell being glucose, methionine, pAB, and pantothenate. Outside the erythrocyte, the plasmodium not only fails to multiply but rapidly dies unless supplied with a variety of supportive substances that it previously obtained from the red cell (Table II-1), and even then its activity only adumbrates that of the intracellular parasite. If we consider the parasitized erythrocyte as the true reproductive unit of the blood stage of the malarial parasite, the plasmodium itself clearly furnishes the enzymic machinery necessary for multiplication, while the erythrocyte furnishes the only environment in which this machinery can function efficiently. Since most other organisms carry out the same biosynthetic reactions in much simpler environments, we may conclude that there are certain defects in the biosynthetic apparatus of the malarial parasite that prevent its functioning extracellularly.

The Defect in Coenzyme A Synthesis

When Trager (1952, 1954) found that Co A, but not pantothenate, greatly lengthened the extracellular survival of *P. lophurae*, he hypothesized that this organism was unable to synthesize Co A and that it was normally synthesized and supplied to the parasite by its host. Trager further pointed out that if this was true, then the inability to make Co A was a major biochemical lesion tending to restrict plasmodia to life within other cells.

The biosynthetic pathway leading first to pantothenate and thence to Co A is shown in Diagram II-3 (see Hoagland and Novelli, 1954, for details). Many bacteria can synthesize Co A *de novo* from simple carbon and nitrogen sources; some require only β-alanine or pantoic acid; and others, such as the lactobacilli, can utilize only the intact pantothenate mole-

DIAGRAM II-3

Biosynthesis of Coenzyme A

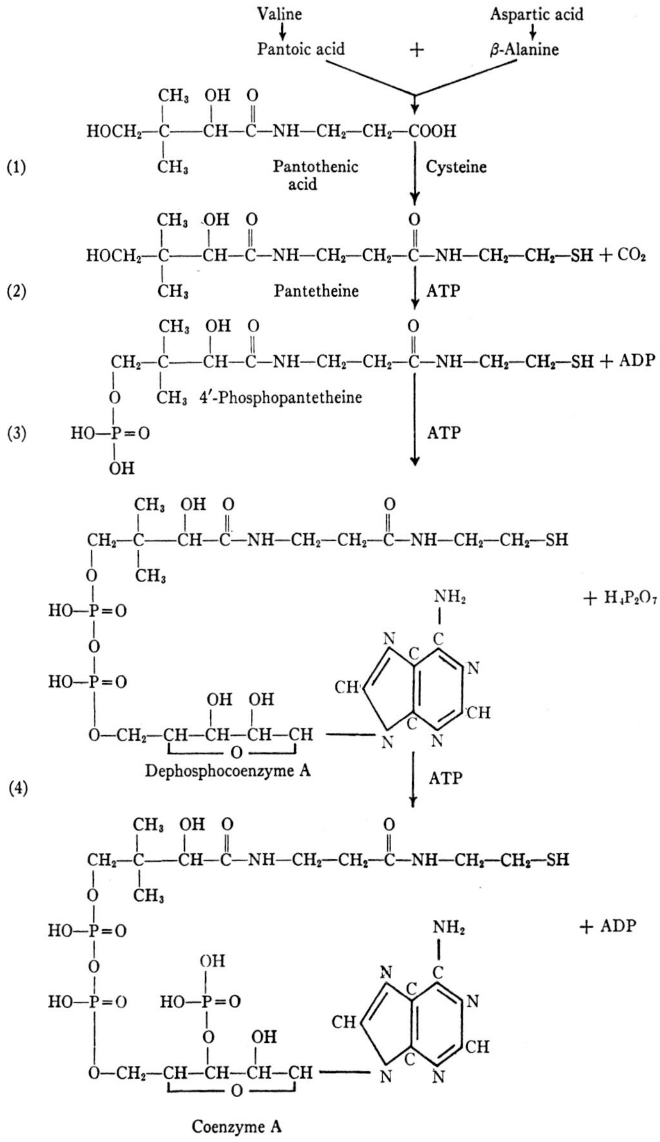

```
        Valine                          Aspartic acid
          ↓                                   ↓
      Pantoic acid         +              β-Alanine
```

(1)
$$HOCH_2-\underset{\underset{CH_3}{|}}{\overset{\overset{CH_3}{|}}{C}}-\overset{\overset{OH}{|}}{CH}-\overset{\overset{O}{\|}}{C}-NH-CH_2-CH_2-COOH$$

Pantothenic acid

Cysteine ↓

(2)
$$HOCH_2-\underset{\underset{CH_3}{|}}{\overset{\overset{CH_3}{|}}{C}}-\overset{\overset{OH}{|}}{CH}-\overset{\overset{O}{\|}}{C}-NH-CH_2-CH_2-\overset{\overset{O}{\|}}{C}-NH-CH_2-CH_2-SH + CO_2$$

Pantetheine   ATP ↓

(3)
$$CH_2-\underset{\underset{CH_3}{|}}{\overset{\overset{CH_3}{|}}{C}}-\overset{\overset{OH}{|}}{CH}-\overset{\overset{O}{\|}}{C}-NH-CH_2-CH_2-\overset{\overset{O}{\|}}{C}-NH-CH_2-CH_2-SH + ADP$$

4'-Phosphopantetheine

$$HO-\overset{\overset{O}{\|}}{P}=O$$
$$OH$$

ATP ↓

(4)

Dephosphocoenzyme A + H₄P₂O₇

ATP ↓

Coenzyme A + ADP

cule. Most animal cells also need pantothenate. One lactobacillus, *Lactobacillus bulgaricus*, must have pantetheine (Craig
and Snell, 1951), while *Acetobacter suboxydans* grows better
on Co A than on pantothenate. Only one organism other than
P. lophurae has been reported to require a form of pantothenate more complex than pantetheine. This is a non-patho-
genic strain of *Treponema pallidum*, the syphilis spirochete,
which must be supplied with either 4-phosphopantetheine or
the coenzyme itself (Steinman *et al.*, 1954). There is thus a
continuous natural spectrum of ability to construct the complex Co A molecule with the obligately intracellular malarial
parasite at the pole of extreme incompetence.

There are at least four steps in the conversion of pantothenate into Co A, and the exact site or sites of the biosynthetic
block(s) in plasmodia are not known. ATP participates in
three of the four steps, once as an adenyl-donating agent and
twice as a phosphorylating agent. One can but wonder
whether perhaps the malarial parasite unnaturally forced
into an extracellular environment is unable to generate or
transfer the high-energy phosphate group of ATP in a normal
fashion. Such speculation suggests that the malarial parasite
itself may be able to synthesize Co A in the red cell and unable to do so outside it. On the other hand, it is equally possible that, as suggested by Trager, the plasmodia are completely without the ability to make Co A either within or
without the erythrocyte. The observation (Trager, 1954) that
parasitized erythrocytes have elevated Co A levels, while the
livers of infected birds have a lessened content of the coenzyme, offers yet a third possibility: the Co A required by
intracellular plasmodia may be synthesized in distant extra-
erythrocytic sites and transported to the parasitized erythrocytes via the blood stream.

Since Co A is required both for the energy-yielding oxidation of glucose via the Krebs cycle and for the synthesis of all

or part of the carbon skeletons of almost all cellular constituents by the addition of 2-carbon units through the acetylating action of acetyl–Co A, an insufficiency of Co A may be expected to lead to grave metabolic disturbances.

The Defect in Carbohydrate Oxidation

Although the malarial parasite within its erythrocyte host competently oxidizes glucose via the Embden-Meyerhof and Krebs cycles, its carbohydrate metabolism becomes seriously deranged when it is freed from the red cell by saponin (Bovarnick, Lindsay, and Hellerman, 1946) or by antiserum and complement (Speck, Moulder, and Evans, 1946). Free parasites convert glucose to lactate at an undiminished or even increased rate but oxidize pyruvate at less than a third the rate exhibited within the erythrocyte host. This rate can be increased 50–75 per cent by the addition of catalytic amounts of a Krebs cycle acid such as malate, ATP, and various coenzymes—DPN and TPN in particular (Speck, Moulder, and Evans, 1946). Still, even with all these additions, which are without effect on pyruvate oxidation in parasitized erythrocytes, free parasites can oxidize pyruvate at only half the rate shown by a comparable number of parasites inside the red cell. There is also a striking qualitative change in glucose and pyruvate metabolism accompanying liberation from the erythrocyte. Acetate is produced by free parasites in large amounts and is not further metabolized. These observations all suggest that the step in glucose breakdown most easily damaged upon release of the parasite from its host is that leading from pyruvate to citrate (Diagram II-4). Acetate accumulation undoubtedly represents the breakdown of a form of active acetate that is formed by the oxidation of pyruvate at a rate faster than it can be removed by condensation with oxalacetate to form citrate. This conclusion finds support in the observation that parasitized erythrocytes, which normally produce no acetate, will form significant amounts when the rate of pyruvate removal is slower than the rate of its formation, as in the oxidation of glucose in the presence of malonate.

There is a striking correlation between the cofactors needed for pyruvate oxidation in free parasites of *P. gallinaceum* and the requirement for survival of free parasites of *P. lophurae*

DIAGRAM II-4

"SENSITIVE" ENZYMIC REACTIONS IN MALARIAL PARASITES

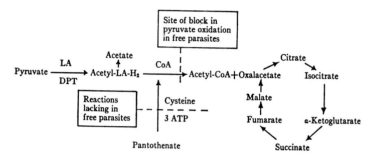

(Table II-1). With the exception of leucovorin and the red cell extract, all the survival-enhancing factors are directly concerned with pyruvate oxidation. The existence of Co A was only suspected at the time that pyruvate oxidation in *P. gallinaceum* was studied, and so we may only speculate on whether its addition would have restored the rate of pyruvate oxidation to the intra-erythrocytic level.

However, Trager's hypothesis that plasmodia are unable to synthesize Co A outside their host cells neatly explains the shift in pattern of carbohydrate metabolism accompanying liberation of the parasite from the erythrocyte (Diagram II-4). Assuming that the details of pyruvate oxidation are the same in plasmodia as in other organisms, pyruvate is bound to a diphosphothiamin-enzyme complex, decarboxylated to acetaldehyde, and transferred to an α-lipoic acid-enzyme complex, in which form it is oxidized to enzyme-bound acetyl-α-lipoic acid. When optimum amounts of Co A are present, as in parasitized erythrocytes, acetyl–Co A is formed and combined with oxalacetate to enter the Krebs cycle as citrate. If Co A is absent or in limiting concentration, acetyl-α-lipoic acid accumulates and breaks down to acetate. Thus the lack of Co A in free parasites logically explains the lessened rate of pyruvate oxidation via the Krebs cycle, the accumulation of acetate, and the requirement of a variety of substances known to facilitate pyruvate oxidation for the extra-erythrocytic survival of plasmodia. It is difficult to escape the conclusion that the inability of plasmodia to synthesize Co A extracellularly results in extensive dislocations in glucose metabolism, which in turn contribute heavily to the restriction of the malarial parasite to an intracellular habitat.

The Defect in Folic Acid Coenzyme Synthesis

p-Aminobenzoic acid (Anfinsen *et al.*, 1946) and pteroylglutamic acid (Glenn and Manwell, 1956) favor multiplication of plasmodia inside red cells but are without effect on their extracellular survival. Leucovorin, which is probably closer in structure to the active coenzyme form of folic acid, does, however, have a definitely favorable action on extracellular survival (Trager, 1958). Since it is unlikely that the red cell can convert *p*AB to pteroylglutamic acid, this synthesis is probably accomplished by the parasite. On the other hand, animal cells can make leucovorin and coenzyme forms of folic acid from pteroylglutamic acid, and Trager (1959, 1961) has suggested that the infected red cell and not the parasite makes the coenzyme forms of folic acid required for plasmodial growth.

The Possibility of a Permeability "Defect"

Table II-1 illustrates a remarkable property of free, extracellular malarial parasites—their ability to take up a number of highly polar substances to which ordinary cells are almost completely impermeable. ATP, the pyridine nucleotides, diphosphothiamin, Co A, and the acids of the tricarboxylic acid cycle nearly always fail to penetrate intact cells; yet they obviously get inside free malarial parasites, as shown by their effects on survival and the oxidation of pyruvate.

This ability to take up large, complex, and metabolically active molecules is clearly of great advantage in intracellular existence. In fact, without this ability, little is gained by living inside a cell in preference to outside. Thus, it seems reasonable that, in the course of evolutionary adaptation to life inside the red cell, the malarial parasite may have lost many of the active transport systems regulating passage of molecules in both directions across its cell membrane and have become freely permeable to all sorts of molecules which it derives directly from its host and no longer bothers to make for itself.

If this is true, then when the plasmodium is unnaturally thrust into an extracellular environment low in these substances, by virtue of the same properties of free permeability so valuable inside the host cell, it cannot hold on to its stores of cofactors, such as ATP and Co A, and they quickly diffuse away. This seems to be very much like what happens when malarial parasites are released extracellularly. It explains their need for so many polar cofactors that are generally without effect on intact cells and offers another powerful reason for limiting plasmodia to an intracellular existence.

Conclusions

We have just discussed a number of defects in the metabolic functioning of the malarial parasite that may be of importance in explaining why it is an obligate intracellular parasite. It is surely not coincidental that all these biochemical lesions are connected more or less directly with the breakdown of glucose, for this is the only phase of carbohydrate metabolism of which we have any sort of satisfactory understanding. There is no reason to suppose that similar shortcomings in the handling of lipid, protein, and nucleic acid will not be revealed by more intensive studies of these aspects of plasmodial metabolism.

We may conclude that the malarial parasite is an organism with wide metabolic capability but with a comparative handful of restrictive enzymic peculiarities which it has acquired in the course of long and successful adaptation to intracellular life.

REFERENCES

ALLISON, A. C. 1954. Brit. M. J., 1:290–94.

ANFINSEN, C. B., GEIMAN, Q. M., McKEE, R. W., ORMSBEE, R. A., and BALL, E. G. 1946. J. Exper. Med., 84:607–21.

BALL, E. G., McKEE, R. W., ANFINSEN, C. B., CRUZ, W. O., and GEIMAN, Q. M. 1948. J. Biol. Chem., 175:547–71.

BOVARNICK, M. R., LINDSAY, A., and HELLERMAN, L. 1946. J. Biol. Chem., 163:535–51.

BROWN, W. H. 1911. J. Exper. Med., 13:290–99.

CHRISTOPHERS, S. R., and FULTON, J. D. 1938. Ann. Trop. Med. Parasitol., 32:43–75.

CLARKE, D. H. 1952a. J. Exper. Med., 96:439–49.

———. 1952b. *Ibid.*, pp. 451–63.

COOK, L., GRANT, P. T., and KERMACK, W. O. 1961. Exper. Parasitol., 11:372–79.

CRAIG, J. A., and SNELL, E. E. 1951. J. Bact., 61:283–91.

DEEGAN, T., and MAEGRAITH, B. G. 1956. Ann. Trop. Med. Parasitol., 50:194–211.

FULTON, J. D., and FLEWETT, T. H. 1956. Trans. Roy. Soc. Trop. Med. Hyg., 50:150–56.

FULTON, J. D., and GRANT, P. T. 1956. Biochem. J., 63:274–82.

GLENN, S., and MANWELL, R. D. 1956. Exper. Parasitol., 5:22–33.

GROMAN, N. B. 1951. J. Infect. Dis., 88:126–50.

HOAGLAND, M. B., and NOVELLI, G. D. 1954. J. Biol. Chem., 174:37–44.

INGRAM, V. M. 1959. Brit. M. Bull., 15:27–32.

KEILIN, D., and HARTREE, E. F. 1947. Biochem. J., 41:503–6.

LEHMAN, H. 1959. Brit. M. Bull., 15:40–46.

LEWERT, R. M. 1952a. J. Infect. Dis., 91:125–44.

———. 1952b. *Ibid.*, pp. 180–83.

McKEE, R. W., and GEIMAN, Q. M. 1948. Fed. Proc., 7:172.

McKee, R. W., Geiman, Q. M., and Cobbey, T. S., Jr. 1947. Fed. Proc., 6:276.

McKee, R. W., Ormsbee, R. A., Anfinsen, C. B., Geiman, Q. M., and Ball, E. G. 1946. J. Exper. Med., 84:569–82.

Morrison, D. B., and Jeskey, H. A. 1947. Fed. Proc., 6:279.

———. 1948. J. Nat. Malaria Soc., 7:259–64.

Moulder, J. W., and Evans, E. A., Jr. 1946. J. Biol. Chem., 164:145–57.

Pauling, L., Itano, H. A., Singer, S. J., and Wells, I. C. 1949. Science, 110:543–48.

Rollo, I. M. 1955. Brit. J. Pharm. Chemotherap., 10:208–14.

Rudzinska, M. A., and Trager, W. 1957. J. Protozoöl., 4:190–99.

———. 1959. J. Biophys. Biochem. Cytol., 6:103–12.

Silverman, M., Ceithaml, J., Taliaferro, L. G., and Evans, E. A., Jr. 1944. J. Infect. Dis., 75:212–30.

Sinton, J. A., and Ghosh, B. N. 1934. Record Malaria Survey India, 4:205–21.

Speck, J. F., and Evans, E. A., Jr. 1945. J. Biol. Chem., 159:71–81.

Speck, J. F., Moulder, J. W., and Evans, E. A., Jr. 1946. J. Biol. Chem., 164:119–44.

Steinman, H. G., Oyama, V. L., and Schulze, H. O. 1954. Fed. Proc., 13:512.

Trager, W. 1941. J. Exper. Med., 74:441–61.

———. 1943. *Ibid.*, 77:411–20.

———. 1947. J. Parasitol., 33:345–50.

———. 1950. J. Exper. Med., 92:349–66.

———. 1952. *Ibid.*, 96:465–76.

———. 1954. J. Protozoöl., 1:231–37.

———. 1958. J. Exper. Med., 108:753–72.

———. 1959. Exper. Parasitol., 8:265–73.

———. 1961. *Ibid.*, 11:298–304.

Wendel, W. B. 1943. J. Biol. Chem., 148:21–34.

Whitfield, P. R. 1953a. Australian J. Biol. Sc., 6:235–43.

———. 1953b. *Ibid.*, pp. 591–96.

CHAPTER III

The Rickettsiae

If malaria wins first place as the most destructive infectious disease, then, according to its official biographer (Zinsser, 1935), typhus runs a close second. Typhus is the most notorious disease caused by the second group of obligate intracellular parasites that we are going to consider. These are the rickettsiae, the etiologic agents of a number of widely occurring and severe infections—the typhus fevers, the spotted fevers, scrub typhus, and Q fever (Table III-1). In appearance, all these micro-organisms are very much alike—they look just like very small bacteria (Fig. III-1). As we shall see, the rickettsiae also behave very much like bacteria and are sequestered into a distinct group mainly because they grow only inside living cells and have never been cultivated on artificial media.

Like malarial parasites, rickettsiae parasitize both vertebrate and invertebrate hosts, but parasitic cycles in this group of organisms show much wider variation, and alternation of hosts is not always required for survival of the species (Table III-1). Zinsser (1935) and others have suggested that the ancestral rickettsiae were parasites of arthropods because intracellular organisms superficially resembling rickettsiae have been found in many different kinds of arthropods, but only a few of these arthropod parasites have been well characterized, and the only one used in metabolic studies (Suitor and Weiss, 1961) differs from rickettsiae in several important respects. However, with the reservation

43

that not all small intracellular arthropod parasites may be rickettsiae, the idea of an arthropod origin for the pathogenic rickettsiae is a sound one. The rickettsiae of the spotted fever group may still be close to this postulated primitive state. These micro-organisms are primarily parasites of various species of ticks found in both the New and the Old World. They do not kill their hosts and are passed through unending generations of ticks by egg transmission. Man and other animals contract spotted fever only when they are bitten by infected ticks, an event of absolutely no importance in the survival of the spotted fever rickettsiae

TABLE III-1

MAJOR RICKETTSIAL DISEASES, THEIR CAUSATIVE
AGENTS AND MODES OF TRANSMISSION

Disease in Man	Causative Agent	Mode of Transmission
Epidemic typhus......	*R. prowazeki*	... Man→Louse→Man→Louse ...
Murine typhus........	*R. mooseri*	... Rat→Rat→Rat→Rat→Rat ... flea flea ↘ Man
Rocky Mountain spotted fever, boutonneuse fever, other spotted fevers.............	*R. rickettsii*	... Tick→Tick→Tick→Tick ... ↘ ↘ Dog Man ↘ Man
Scrub typhus (tsutsugamushi fever)........	*R. tsutsugamushi*	... Mite→Field→Mite→Field ... mouse ↘ mouse Man
Rickettsial pox........	*R. akari*	... Mite→House→Mite→House ... mouse ↘ mouse Man
Q fever..............	*Coxiella burnetii*	... Tick→Small→Tick→Cattle ... mammal air- ↘ borne Man

in nature. Murine typhus—the endemic flea-borne typhus fever of the southern United States and Mexico—has a parasitic cycle which may resemble that of the first rickettsiae to grow regularly in mammalian hosts. The normal arthropod host is the rat flea, and the normal mammalian host is the rat. Man is merely an accidental host who becomes infected when a typhus-bearing flea bites him instead of another rat. In epidemic louse-borne typhus of world-wide distribution, man himself has become the definitive mammalian host, and his inseparable companion—the human body louse—the insect vector. Epidemic typhus is thus a peculiarly human disease.

Again, as with malarial parasites, it would be of immense interest to compare the biochemical behavior of rickettsiae grown in their arthropod hosts, on the one hand, and their mammalian hosts, on the other, but practical considerations have again smothered theoretical desirabilities, and biochemical investigations on rickettsiae have all been performed with rickettsiae grown in a vertebrate host.

Almost all biochemical work has been carried out with the two varieties of typhus rickettsiae, *Rickettsia prowazeki* and *R. mooseri*, but limited studies with *R. rickettsii* and *Coxiella burnetii* show no great divergence in metabolic patterns within the rickettsia family. Thus we feel reasonably safe in applying results obtained with one agent to the explanation of the behavior of another.

GROWTH, MORPHOLOGY, AND CHEMICAL COMPOSITION
Growth of Rickettsiae in Experimental Systems

Rickettsiae have been successfully cultivated in small laboratory animals and in lice in quantities large enough to be used as vaccines, but when Cox (1938) discovered that they could be easily grown in large numbers in the yolk sacs of chick embryos, his procedure rapidly replaced all others in the laboratory cultivation of large numbers of rickettsiae. We shall return to yolk-sac cultivation when considering methods for preparing purified rickettsial suspensions for metabolic investigations.

While the yolk sac is best for growing large numbers of rickettsiae, details of this growth may be more easily studied in infected cell cultures. Perhaps the most extensive study is that of the group at the Walter Reed Army Institute on the growth of *R. tsutsugamushi* in various cell lines of mouse origin. When highly infective rickettsiae were mixed with living cells, the rickettsiae rapidly penetrated the host cells, and, with high inocula, almost all cells in the cultures became infected in 1–2 hours (Cohn *et al.*, 1959). Anything that reduced the metabolic activity of the rickettsiae reduced their ability to infect cells in culture. Killed organisms did not get inside host cells at all. Killing the host cells also reduced penetration practically to zero. The relation of rickettsial metabolism to absorption on and penetration into the host cell will be considered after we have discussed the metabolic properties of these micro-organisms.

Once within the host cell, the rickettsiae reproduced by binary fission (Schaechter *et al.*, 1957a). Their number increased about threefold every 24 hours. Within a few days they became visible as large clusters of organisms growing in the cytoplasm in regions surrounding the nucleus. This is a comparatively slow growth rate as compared with bacteria. Rickettsiae of the spotted fever group are regularly found in nuclei of infected cells, but the other agents do not invade the nucleus. Multiplication occurred only when the mouse cells were suspended in a complete medium capable of supporting active cell proliferation (Hopps *et al.*, 1959). This observation contradicts older, less carefully controlled studies, which had led to the widely quoted conclusion that rickettsiae grow best in dead or dying cells. In the experience of Hopps *et al.*, when the cells were suspended in maintenance medium, the rickettsiae not only failed to multiply but actually died off gradually.

There seems to be no definite growth cycle in rickettsial infections as in malaria or in infections with the psittacosis group agents. Multiplication by binary fission appears to continue until the cell is filled with rickettsiae. The cell then bursts and releases its contents into the surrounding medium.

Morphology

Rickettsiae stain readily with basic stains, such as Machiavello's, Giemsa's, and Castenada's. Stained smears from infected tissues show a variety of rickettsial bodies ranging from spheres about 0.3 μ in diameter to long rods up to 2 μ in length. The predominant forms are usually short rods about 0.3 $\times$ 1.0 μ in size. Ris and Fox (1949) have shown that the cytology of rickettsiae is very similar to that of bacteria. When unwashed rickettsiae were stained with the basic stain methyl green–pyronin, they stained uniformly red with the pyronin portion of the reagent, indicating the presence of RNA throughout the cytoplasm. Treatment with ribonuclease practically abolished the pyronin staining and left one or more discrete bodies staining purple with the methyl green. This dye has a strong affinity for DNA, and it is highly probable that these ribonuclease-resistant bodies were DNA-containing structures corresponding to the nuclear structures or chromatinic bodies of bacteria. Mere washing with physiological saline also greatly reduced the pyronin staining. Ris and Fox interpreted this as meaning that the RNA was washed out.

Electron microscopy confirms the resemblance of rickettsial morphology to that of bacteria. Purified suspensions of rickettsiae dried directly on specimen grids with or without metal shadowing (Fig. III-1) showed bodies with limiting membranes surrounding a granular cytoplasm containing one or more dense central bodies (Plotz *et al.*, 1943; Ris and Fox, 1949; Kausche and Sheris, 1951; Wissig *et al.*, 1956). The spherical bodies usually had only one dense body, while the rod-shaped ones frequently had two or more. Wissig *et al.* (1956) examined thin sections of yolk sac infected with the agents of murine typhus and scrub typhus (Fig. III-2), while Stoker *et al.* (1956) sectioned pellets of purified *C. burnetii* (Fig. III-3). Both kinds of sectioned material again indicated that rickettsiae had a limiting membrane and a dense central body surrounded by a less dense cytoplasm. Stoker *et al.* felt that the central body might be an elongated and twisted strand.

Chemical Composition

Completely satisfactory chemical analyses on purified rickettsiae are not available. Cohen and Chargaff (1944), Tovarnickij *et al.* (1946) and Cohen (1950) found protein, carbohydrate, neutral fat, and phospholipid in purified preparations of *R. prowazeki*. Unfortunately, these studies were made before it was realized that rickettsiae leak many of their cell constituents when washed in salt solutions at room temperature. Both groups, for example, found DNA but no RNA, while later investigators (Cohn *et al.*, 1958), using improved purification methods which minimize leakage, found three times as much RNA as DNA in *R. mooseri*.

Smith and Stoker (1951) studied the amino acids and nucleic acids of *C. burnetii* purified by rather drastic means which probably resulted in some leakage of RNA. Most of the common amino acids were present, together with 9.7 per cent DNA and 4.3 per cent RNA. Their analysis

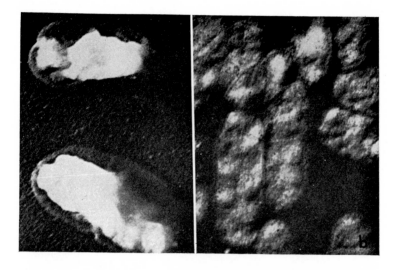

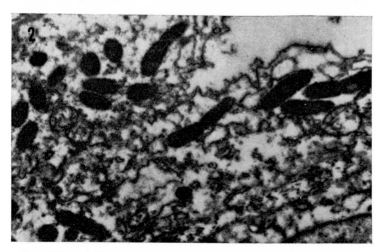

Figs. III-1 and III-2.—From Wissig *et al.* (1956), reproduced by permission of the authors and the *American Journal of Pathology*. Fig. III-1: Electron micrographs of washed suspensions of *R. mooseri*. *a*, Dried on the specimen grid and shadowed with chromium. 50,000✕. *b*, Fixed with osmic acid in suspension and then dried and shadowed with gold-manganin. 50,000✕. Fig. III-2: Electron micrograph of osmium-fixed thin section of yolk-sac cell infected with *R. mooseri*. 21,000✕.

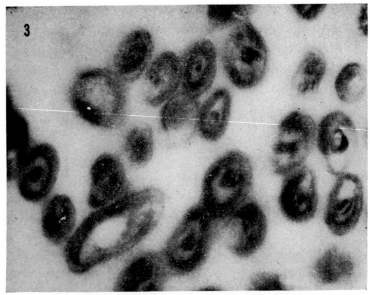

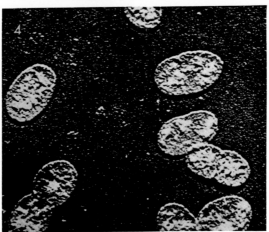

Figs. III-3 and III-4.—Fig. III-3: Electron micrograph of thin section of osmium-fixed pellet of purified *C. burnetii*. From Stoker *et al.* (1956). Reproduced by permission of the authors and the *Journal of General Microbiology*. 64,000×. Fig. III-4: Electron micrograph of cell walls of *R. mooseri*, fixed with osmium tetroxide, dried in air, and shadowed with uranium. From Schaechter *et al.* (1957). Reproduced by permission of the authors and the *Journal of Bacteriology*. 20,000×.

of the base content of *C. burnetii* DNA is compared in Table III-2 with similar data for *R. prowazeki* obtained by Wyatt and Cohen (1952). It is of considerable interest to note that the base ratios in the two organisms are clearly different. Price (1953*a*) found both DNA and RNA in *R. rickettsii*.

Schaechter *et al.* (1957*b*) prepared cell walls from *R. mooseri* by treating purified rickettsiae with deoxycholate (Fig. III-4). These structures obviously correspond to the limiting membranes seen in electron micrographs of whole organisms and are responsible for their shape and size. In chemical

TABLE III-2

BASE COMPOSITION OF DEOXYRIBONUCLEIC ACID OF
R. prowazeki and *C. burnetii*

ORGANISM	MOLES PER CENT BASE			
	Adenine	Thymine	Guanine	Cytosine
R. prowazeki.......	35.7	31.8	17.1	15.4
C. burnetii	29.5	26.0	22.5	22.0

composition, they resembled the cell walls of bacteria, in that they were composed mainly of amino acids and polysaccharides. However, they did not contain such distinctive bacterial cell-wall constituents as diaminopimelic acid or muramic acid, and they did contain glucuronic acid, which does not usually occur in cell walls of bacteria. Allison and Perkins (1960) prepared cell walls of *C. burnetii* by the method of Schaechter *et al.* and found a similar composition, with the important exception that a positive test for muramic acid was obtained. Since muramic acid (3-0-α-carboxyethyl-glucosamine) has not been found except in bacteria and blue-green algae (Salton, 1960), this is a most important observation.

In general, the scanty chemical evidence confirms the morphologic impression that rickettsiae are very much like bacteria.

Susceptibility to Chemotherapeutic Agents

Rickettsial multiplication is inhibited by a number of antibiotics. The tetracyclines are effective inhibitors of all rickettsial species, while erythromycin and chloramphenicol are highly active against all except the agent of Q fever (Ormsbee *et al.*, 1955). Penicillin has only slight activity. In these respects, the rickettsiae again resemble bacteria. However, they are not inhibited by sulfonamides but are, instead, inhibited by pAB, the essential metabolite whose functioning is interfered with by sulfonamides in sulfa-sensitive micro-organisms (Greiff *et al.*, 1944; Hamilton *et al.*, 1945). Since the rickettsiostatic action of pAB is reversed by p-hydroxybenzoic acid (Snyder and Davis, 1951; Takemori and Kitaoka, 1952), it is probable that the p-hydroxy compound is essential for rickettsial multiplication and that its normal functioning is prevented by excess pAB.

METABOLIC PATHWAYS

We have seen in the preceding chapter how studies on metabolic pathways and nutritional requirements of malarial parasites reinforced and complemented each other. A similar situation exists in biochemical investigations on the rickettsiae. Here the two principal areas of study have been metabolic pathways and factors affecting the stability of rickettsial properties, such as infectivity, toxicity, and hemolytic activity. Considerable success has been achieved in maintaining and restoring these activities in purified rickettsiae incubated in vitro, and this achievement represents the first step toward eventual culture of these organisms in artificial media in the absence of other living cells.

We shall again take up, first, the nature of the metabolic reactions occurring in rickettsiae, although this discussion will inevitably involve some of the investigations on in vitro stability.

Preparation of Purified Rickettsial Suspensions

Malarial parasites have relatively high metabolic rates and grow in biochemically sluggish cells, so that their metabolism may be measured while they are still inside their host cells. When the plasmodia are freed from their erythrocyte hosts and studied in the free state, the presence of residual host material in the free parasite preparations is no serious problem. In contrast, the rate of rickettsial respiration and the ratio of rickettsial mass to host-cell mass are both so low that infected cells show no increased metabolic activity (Bozeman *et al.*, 1956). Thus we cannot study the metabolism of rickettsiae growing intracellularly and are forced to extrapolate this behavior within host cells from the metabolic activities expressed by free rickettsiae.

In preparing rickettsial suspensions suitable for metabolic study, the investigator must steer a perilous course between the Scylla of host contamination and the Charybdis of rickettsial inactivation. The difficulties in distinguishing between host and rickettsial enzymes make the removal of host contaminants of critical importance, but rickettsiae are none too stable in crude suspensions and rapidly become even less so as stabilizing host proteins are removed in the course of purification. The successful elucidation of many aspects of rickettsial metabolism in the last ten years has been due in large part to the satisfactory solution of these inherently antagonistic problems.

Diagram III-1 shows the major steps in a typical preparation of metabolically active rickettsiae relatively free of contaminating host material. Infected chick-embryo yolk sac has been the almost universal starting material (Cox, 1938). The general procedure has been to subject the yolk-sac emulsions to a series of differential centrifugations, with the rickettsiae appearing in the sediment at high speed and in the supernatant at low speed. Since the rickettsiae are appreciably sedimented in all but the lowest fields, the efficiency

DIAGRAM III-1

Isolation of Purified Rickettsiae from Chick-Embryo Yolk Sac

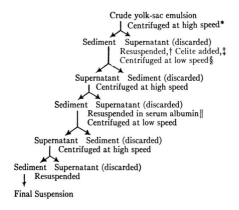

Crude yolk-sac emulsion
Centrifuged at high speed*

Sediment   Supernatant (discarded)
Resuspended,† Celite added,‡
Centrifuged at low speed§

Supernatant   Sediment (discarded)
Centrifuged at high speed

Sediment   Supernatant (discarded)
Resuspended in serum albumin‖
Centrifuged at low speed

Supernatant   Sediment (discarded)
Centrifuged at high speed

Sediment   Supernatant (discarded)
Resuspended

Final Suspension

* 3,500 rcf for 60 minutes.
† Typical suspending media:

Salt Medium	Sucrose Medium
0.126 M KCl	0.225 M sucrose
0.0018 M NaCl	0.0016 M KH_2PO_4
0.0106 M Na_2PHO_4	0.0086 M K_3HPO_4
0.0012 M KH_2PO_4	pH 7.5
pH 7.5	

‡ 1 gm. Celite (Johns-Manville Hyflo Supercel) per 6 gm. yolk sac.
§ 500 rcf for 30 minutes.
‖ 6 per cent bovine serum albumin, 1 ml. per gm. yolk sac.

of the low-speed removal of host material has been increased by adding substances that flocculate it and bolster its sedimentation. Celite—a diatomaceous earth—was introduced for this purpose by Fulton and Begg (1946) and Shepard and Topping (1947) in the preparation of rickettsial antigens and was used by Bovarnick and Snyder (1949) in the first preparation of metabolically active rickettsiae. Bovarnick and Miller (1950) removed still more yolk-sac material from Celite-treated suspensions by flocculation with serum albumin. Purified preparations made with Celite and serum albumin have proved satisfactory for most metabolic studies, but further separation of rickettsiae from host contaminants can be achieved by digestion with trypsin (Wisseman *et al.*, 1951) or by precipitation with antiserum against normal yolk-sac antigens (Price, 1953*a;* Karp, 1954; Paretsky *et al.*, 1958). When purifications such as these were carried out at 0° C. with the use of media of suitable composition (to be discussed later), 50–75 per cent of the original rickettsiae were recovered, with their original infectivity, toxicity, and hemolytic activity still apparently intact.

The chief criteria for the freedom of purified suspensions from normal yolk-sac components have been morphologic and immunologic: the absence of recognizable particles of host origin in electron micrographs and the absence of host antigens as determined by complement fixation with antiserum against normal yolk sac (Hopps *et al.*, 1956). It is generally agreed that a small amount of host material remains in the best preparations. In order to determine whether an enzymic activity observed in a purified suspension is attributable to the rickettsiae or to residual host material, it has been customary to prepare normal yolk-sac preparations by taking uninfected yolk sac through all the steps of the rickettsial purification procedure and to test these normal particle suspensions for the activity in question.

Oxidation of Glutamate

Rickettsiae possess a highly distinctive respiratory metabolism. They fail to attack glucose, glucose-6-phosphate, or lactate either aerobically or anaerobically (Bovarnick and Snyder, 1949). They are also unable to oxidize all the amino acids except one, glutamic acid, which appears to be the chief energy source (Bovarnick and Snyder, 1949;

Bovarnick and Miller, 1950; Wisseman *et al.*, 1951, 1952; Price, 1953*a;* Karp, 1954; Paretsky *et al.*, 1958).

Glutamate oxidation was the first independent metabolic activity found in rickettsiae (Bovarnick and Snyder, 1949); hence early workers spent considerable time in obtaining evidence to show that the glutamate oxidation observed in rickettsial suspensions was a true rickettsial function and not due to carry-over of host enzymes. Bovarnick and Snyder demonstrated that normal yolk-sac preparations did not consume oxygen in the presence of glutamate and that the rate of glutamate oxidation in rickettsial suspensions was roughly proportional to their mouse toxicity (a good measure of the concentration of viable organisms present—see later sections). This relation held for both epidemic and murine typhus preparations. Wisseman *et al.* (1951) confirmed these observations with murine typhus rickettsiae, while Karp (1954) showed that treatment of purified rickettsiae with antiserum against normal yolk sac removed a number of enzymic activities but left the rate of glutamate oxidation unchanged. She also showed that rickettsial preparations from mouse lung oxidized glutamate at the same rate as those made from yolk sac. All these observations establish beyond any reasonable doubt that rickettsiae possess enzymes for the aerobic oxidation of glutamate.

Bovarnick and Miller (1950) found that the chief products of glutamate oxidation were ammonia, carbon dioxide, and aspartate. This suggested that glutamate was oxidized to α-ketoglutarate, which could then be either transaminated to aspartate or further oxidized (Diagram III-2). We shall consider rickettsial transaminations a little later and concentrate on that portion of the glutamate that was further oxidized. Bovarnick and Miller (1950) also found that α-ketoglutarate, succinate, and pyruvate were oxidized by rickettsiae, but at much slower rates than glutamate. This raised the possibility that glutamate was oxidized via a Krebs tricarboxylic acid cycle (Diagram III-3).

Wisseman *et al.* (1952) continued the investigation of pathways of glutamate oxidation with *R. mooseri* preparations. They found that a-ketoglutarate, succinate, fumarate, malate, oxalacetate, and pyruvate significantly increased the very low endogenous oxygen uptake—again much less than glutamate. However, the tricarboxylic acids of the Krebs cycle gave no evidence of being attacked by the rickettsiae. They then attempted to satisfy the classic requirements for the demonstration of a Krebs cycle for glutamate oxidation (see discussion in chap. ii) with the following results: (1) a-ketoglutarate and ammonia accumulated in the presence of arsenite, a selective inhibitor for a-ketoglutaric dehydrogenase; (2) in the presence of malo-

DIAGRAM III-2

FATE OF GLUTAMATE IN RICKETTSIAE

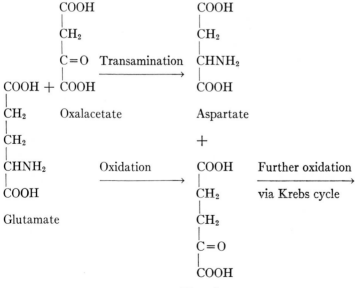

a-Ketoglutarate

57

nate, the accumulation of traces of succinate could be demonstrated by a microspectrophotometric method; (3) the 2,4-dinitrophenylhydrazones of α-ketoglutarate, oxalacetate, and pyruvate were isolated; (4) aspartate accumulated, as already shown by Bovarnick and Miller (1950). Attempts to demonstrate citrate accumulations in the presence of *trans*-aconitate and fluoroacetate—both inhibitors of isocitric dehydrogenase—were unsuccessful.

DIAGRAM III-3

THE KREBS TRICARBOXYLIC ACID CYCLE IN RICKETTSIAE

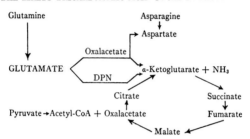

Price (1953a) reported in a preliminary paper that spotted fever rickettsiae oxidized glutamate, pyruvate, α-ketoglutarate, succinate, fumarate, malate, and oxalacetate. Succinate accumulated during oxidation of glutamate, and citrate was formed from pyruvate and oxalacetate in the presence of ATP, Co A, α-lipoic acid, and glutathione. Unfortunately, the details of these experiments have never been published.

Paretsky *et al.* (1958) found that *C. burnetii* formed citrate from either acetate or acetyl-phosphate and that DPN, ATP, Co A, and oxalacetate were required for the reaction.

Taken together, all these observations are very strong arguments for the oxidation of glutamate via a Krebs tricarboxylic acid cycle, although the existence of such an oxidative mechanism in rickettsiae cannot be regarded as strictly proved. The dicarboxylic acids of the Krebs cycle are oxidized at much slower rates than glutamate, and the tricarboxylic acids of the citrate family are not oxidized at all. However, as first suggested by Bovarnick and Miller (1950), this inertness may only reflect the relative impermeability of intact rickettsiae to the acids of the Krebs cycle. Such impermeability would explain why freezing and thawing, which reduce viability, increase the activity of succinate in promoting oxygen uptake (Bovarnick and Snyder, 1949) and of oxalacetate in increasing transamination (Bovarnick and Miller, 1950; Hopps *et al.*, 1956).

Oxidation of Pyruvate

A number of workers have observed that rickettsiae consume oxygen in the presence of pyruvate, but only Bovarnick and Miller (1950) have studied its oxidation in any detail. They found that 1–2 moles of oxygen are consumed for every mole of pyruvate which disappears and that the R.Q. of pyruvate oxidation is 1.3–1.4. This indicates that pyruvate is oxidized beyond the acetate stage, presumably via acetyl-Co A and the Krebs cycle.

Transamination

The existence of transaminases in rickettsiae was first suspected by Bovarnick and Miller (1950) when they found that much more glutamate disappeared than could be accounted for by the ammonia liberated. This missing glutamate ammonia was quantitatively accounted for as aspartate. Bovarnick and Miller assumed that part of the glutamate was oxidized to oxalacetate, which then transaminated with unchanged glutamate to form aspartate and α-ketoglutarate (Diagram III-2). Addition of oxalacetate increased the rate of aspartate accumulation (Bovarnick and Miller, 1950;

59

Hopps *et al.*, 1956), particularly when the rickettsial suspension was frozen and thawed to increase its permeability to oxalacetate. This treatment destroyed viability and the glutamate oxidase system but left the rickettsial transaminase unaffected. Normal yolk-sac preparations showed a slight transaminase activity, but with these preparations there was no enhancement of the oxalacetate effect by freezing and thawing.

Transaminases other than the glutamate-oxalacetate enzyme have not been found in rickettsiae.

Electron Transport

Various observations gave early indication that electron transport in rickettsiae was mediated by respiratory enzymes analogous to those of other organisms. The reactivation of several rickettsial activities by DPN (see later section) implicated pyridinoprotein enzymes; the presence of large concentrations of riboflavin (Kleinschmidt *et al.*, 1956) suggested the possibility of flavoprotein catalysis; and the inhibition of glutamate oxidation by cyanide (Wisseman *et al.*, 1951) indicated the functioning of heavy-metal enzymes.

Hayes *et al.* (1957) sought more direct evidence as to the nature of electron-transport systems in rickettsiae by applying the sensitive spectrophotometric methods developed by Chance (1952) for the study of oxidations in higher organisms to the investigation of glutamate oxidation in *R. mooseri*. They obtained a difference spectrum (reduced *minus* oxidized forms of the respiratory pigments) for glutamate oxidation, which corresponded to the absorption maxima and minima for cytochrome a or a_1, cytochrome b_1, and flavoprotein. This constitutes direct evidence for the functioning of cytochromes and flavoproteins in the transport of electrons from glutamate to molecular oxygen. Very high cell densities were necessary to demonstrate this difference spectrum, showing that the concentrations of the enzymes involved were very low, several fold lower than the corresponding concentrations in common aerobic bacteria.

Oxidative Phosphorylation

Bovarnick and Miller (1950) and Price (1953a) found that phosphate was necessary for an optimal rate of glutamate oxidation, and Price briefly reported that inorganic phosphorus was esterified into organic linkage during the oxidation of glutamate by spotted fever rickettsiae.

However, Bovarnick (1956) was the first to give detailed evidence for oxidative phosphorylation in rickettsiae. When *R. prowazeki* oxidized glutamate in the presence of ADP,

DIAGRAM III-4

OXIDATIVE PHOSPHORYLATION IN RICKETTSIAE
(Measurement by Use of the Hexokinase System)

$$\text{Glutamate} + \text{P} + \text{ADP} + \text{O}_2 \rightarrow \text{Oxidation} + \text{ATP}$$
$$\text{products}$$

$$\text{ATP} + \text{Glucose} \xrightarrow{\text{Hexokinase}} \text{Glucose-6-P}$$

glucose, and hexokinase, glucose-6-phosphate was formed via the sequence of events shown in Diagram III-4. Maximum phosphorylation required DPN, Co A, and high concentrations of ADP and inorganic phosphate. A maximum of 0.2–0.3 mole of phosphorus was esterified for each mole of oxygen consumed, a P/O ratio in the range usually encountered in oxidative phosphorylation by intact cells. With particularly active preparations, the actual disappearance of inorganic phosphate could be measured, as well as the appearance of glucose-6-phosphate.

Cyanide inhibited glutamate oxidation and reduced glucose-6-phosphate formation to nearly zero. Dinitrophenol inhibited phosphate uptake without interfering with oxygen consumption, a typical decoupling effect such as that encountered in phosphorylating systems in higher organisms.

All these results point to oxidative phosphorylation during the course of glutamate oxidation as the chief energy source for rickettsiae. This indication is borne out by the results of Bovarnick and Allen (1957*b*), which will be discussed in detail under the general subject of inactivation and reactivation. In brief, they found that the presence of an active oxidative phosphorylation was an important (but not the only) factor in the reactivation of rickettsiae after starvation at 36° C.

In Vitro Syntheses

When purified rickettsiae are maintained in vitro under conditions of maximum stability, a small but definite synthesis of protein and lipid may be observed by measuring the uptake of radioactive amino acids and acetate. Killed rickettsiae and normal yolk-sac preparations show no uptake at all.

Uptake of methionine-S^{35} was first observed (Bovarnick *et al.*, 1959), but the incorporation of glycine-1-C^{14} into rickettsial protein was studied in more detail (Bovarnick and Schneider, 1960*a*). They concluded that "many of the requirements for optimal amino acid incorporation by rickettsiae more resemble those shown by isolated cell particulates than those shown by undamaged cells, a resemblance which may be a consequence of the fact that the rickettsiae, like the cell particulates, normally function inside a cell."

First, incorporation is highly dependent on the inorganic and organic composition of the medium in which the rickettsiae are suspended. In this respect, amino acid incorporation is an even more sensitive indicator of rickettsial well-being than infectivity itself, a point to which we shall return in discussing the stability of rickettsiae.

Second, even the very low rate of glycine uptake required the addition of all the naturally occurring amino acids. Since such a low rate of incorporation occurs endogeneously in other cells previously studied, this requirement suggests that rickettsiae have no pool of free amino acids at all, at least during extracellular in vitro incubation.

Third, uptake of glycine by rickettsiae was strongly stimulated by phosphorylated compounds—DPN and Co A in particular. Long-continued uptake required the presence of ribonucleotides, but deoxyribonucleotides were not needed.

Fourth, both exogenous and endogenous supplies of ATP were required. When endogenous ATP was generated by glutamate oxidation, added ATP increased the rate of glycine uptake. However, when intracellular ATP formation was blocked by cyanide or dinitrophenol, addition of ATP to the suspending medium did not restore glycine uptake. This curious dual requirement for ATP also holds for the activity of the rickettsial hemolysin (Bovarnick and Schneider, 1960b); we shall return to it at the close of the chapter.

While it is always difficult to prove that incorporation of an amino acid represents true synthesis, several observations suggest that the rickettsial uptake represents real protein formation. Omission of a single amino acid, such as serine, threonine, or valine, prevented glycine uptake, and glycine incorporation was inhibited by chloramphenicol, a recognized inhibitor of protein synthesis. Dinitrophenol and cyanide also interfered with incorporation.

When acetate-1-C^{14} was substituted for the labeled glycine, it was incorporated into the rickettsial lipids (Bovarnick, 1960). The uptake of acetate was an order of magnitude less than even the low amino acid uptake, possibly because the labeled acetate was diluted intracellularly by the unlabeled acetate formed from glutamate via the Krebs cycle. However, the incorporation of acetate into lipid occurred at measurable rates, and this indicates that rickettsiae, like other cells, synthesize their lipids by condensing two-carbon units derived from acetate, undoubtedly acetyl-Co A.

These uptakes of amino acids and acetate are very small. About a 100 to 1,000 fold increase in incorporation would be needed to double the rickettsial protein or lipid. However, they are most important because they represent the occurrence of energy-requiring synthetic reactions in vitro. If enough of these synthetic reactions can be induced to occur at sufficient rates, then the rickettsiae will surely also grow and multiply in artificial culture. The slow observed synthetic rates may result from the slow growth rates of rickettsiae in vivo, from the damaging of synthetic enzymes during liberation from the cell and subsequent purification, or from a requirement for unsuspected substrates or cofactors.

Factors Affecting the Stability of Rickettsiae in Vitro

When rickettsiae are removed from their host cells and suspended in the simple buffered salt solutions ordinarily used for metabolic studies on bacteria, they rapidly lose their infectivity and a number of other closely associated properties: their ability to oxidize glutamate, their ability to incorporate amino acids and acetate, their toxicity for mice, and their hemolytic action on the erythrocytes of a number of animals. Bovarnick and her associates have systematically studied the effect of a variety of factors on these rickettsial activities. Their investigations have been of great practical value in establishing conditions of maximum stability under which the properties of rickettsiae may be maintained and studied in vitro. Their theoretical value has been even greater, for the establishment of conditions under which more and more rickettsial activities may be preserved for longer and longer periods of extracellular existence is the only rational course toward eventual artificial cultivation of these micro-organisms.

The close association of toxicity, hemolytic activity, respiration, and incorporation with infectivity is shown by the observations that all these properties accompany infectivity during the purification of rickettsiae, cannot be dissociated from the intact organism, and are frequently lost at the same rate as infectivity at low or elevated temperatures. We shall also see that, in general, anything that tends to destroy or to preserve any one of these properties tends to affect the others in the same way. However, these properties can be dissociated. Incorporation of amino acids into rickettsial protein is even more easily abolished than infectivity itself (Bovarnick and Schneider, 1960a), while respiration, hemolytic activity, and toxicity may be demonstrated in the absence of infectivity. These three properties of rickettsiae are very closely associated but may be separated by progressive dosage with ultraviolet light (Allen *et al.*, 1954).

Optimum Conditions for Rickettsial Survival

Metabolic studies on purified rickettsiae required the development of chemically defined suspending media which would maintain infectivity, respiration, and other properties without great loss for several hours at 30°–35° C. Bovarnick *et al.* (1950) found that survival of rickettsiae at these temperatures was best at about pH 7.5 in a medium high in potassium and low in sodium. Survival was strikingly improved by the addition of glutamate and even more improved by the further addition of DPN (Bovarnick *et al.*, 1953). Serum albumin in concentrations of 0.1–1 per cent had a good effect on survival, as did 0.225 M sucrose.

Two commonly used media are described in Diagram III-1. Different species of rickettsiae were of approximately equal stability, with the exception of *C. burnetii*, which was somewhat hardier.

However, even the best media fail to maintain rickettsiae in a condition suitable for biochemical investigation for longer than 24 hours at 0° C. If they are to be kept for longer periods, they may be shell-frozen in glutamate-DPN media containing 0.05–0.225 M sucrose and 4–6 per cent serum albumin, stored at −70° C., and then rapidly thawed without decrease in infectivity, respiration, and associated properties (Bovarnick *et al.*, 1950).

Reversible Inactivation

When typhus rickettsiae were frozen and thawed in isotonic saline instead of sucrose-albumin, all activity was lost upon thawing; but Bovarnick and Allen (1954) discovered that when these apparently dead organisms were incubated at 34° C. for 2–3 hours in a suitable medium, the most important ingredient of which was DPN, there was a marked increase in the ability to oxidize glutamate. Addition of Co A in the presence of DPN further increased the respiratory rate. DPN assays showed that this coenzyme (and presumably Co A as well) was leached out of the cells frozen and thawed in saline. Since DPN and Co A are coenzymes for glutamate oxidation, it was not surprising that they restored glutamate oxidation in coenzyme-depleted cells. However, Bovarnick and Allen made the unexpected and important discovery that mouse toxicity, hemolytic activity, and often infectivity itself were also restored by incubation at 34° C. with DPN and Co A. They termed this phenomenon "reversible inactivation." Bovarnick and Allen (1957*a*) later obtained a more completely reversible type of inactivation by simply holding purified rickettsial suspensions overnight at 0° C. in isotonic salt solution. Upon incubation at 34° C. in the presence of DPN and glutamate, 50–100 per cent of the original infectivity, toxicity, hemolytic activity, and respiration was restored. As in freezing and thawing, holding at 0° C. in salt solutions caused the release of DPN from the rickettsial cells. While DPN dramatically restored the activity of rickettsiae inactivated by standing at 0° C., its presence at 0° C. did not always prevent the loss of activity, and Bovarnick and Allen suggested that factors other than loss of DPN might also be involved.

An entirely different type of reversible inactivation occurred when typhus rickettsiae were incubated at 36° C. in the absence of substrate (Bovarnick and Allen, 1957*b*). Infectivity, toxicity, hemolytic activity, and respiration were rapidly lost, and this loss could largely be prevented by the addition of glutamate, pyruvate, and ATP. However, only glutamate could restore activity once it was lost. Reactivation was most effective at 30° C. and required 2–3 hours for maximum restoration of activity.

Direct assays by the firefly luminescence test showed that rickettsiae oxidizing glutamate contained measurable quantities of ATP (Bovarnick and Allen, 1957*b*). The ATP level dropped to zero during starvation at 36° C. and rose again during incubation with glutamate. In general, anything which tended to lower the ATP content of the rickettsiae also tended to decrease the extent of recovery. For example, the absence of inorganic phosphate or the presence of a decoupling agent, such as dinitrophenol, lessened reactivation. However, the correlation between reactivation of the different rickettsial activities and the presence of oxidative phosphorylation was not complete. Infectivity lost at 36° C. was not restored under any known conditions, while incubation with glutamate at 35° C. instead of 30° C. promoted active phosphorylation but did not restore the activity of either the toxin or the hemolysin. It is therefore evident that still other factors are operative in the preservation and restoration of these three properties of rickettsiae.

Reversible inactivation at 0° and at 36° C. obviously represents two different kinds of damage to rickettisae and two correspondingly different mechanisms of metabolic repair. Inactivation at 0° C. appears to be largely the result of the loss of diffusible cofactors, of which DPN is the most important. Readdition of DPN is followed by more or less equal reactivation of all rickettsial properties studied, although the reactivation is probably far from a simple process, since it is temperature-dependent and requires several hours for completion. Inactivation at 36° C. occurs equally rapidly in the presence or absence of DPN and appears to result from the loss of intracellular ATP. ATP generated by the oxidation of glutamate is more effective than exogenous extracellular ATP. Endogenous ATP both maintains and restores activity, while exogenous ATP can only maintain. This differential behavior is characteristic of rickettsial metabolism and will be considered again later. Although the correlation between restoration of ATP levels and restoration of other rickettsial properties is not complete, the phenomenon of reversible inactivation at elevated temperatures is very important, in that it clearly establishes the vital role of glutamate oxidation and oxidative phosphorylation in the functioning of rickettsiae.

Factors Influencing Incorporation of Amino Acids

With the information provided by the experiments just described, it became possible to devise media which would preserve the infectivity of typhus rickettsiae almost unchanged for as long as 24–48 hours at 30° C. Yet even under these conditions of near-optimum stability, the rickettsiae did not multiply. Therefore, Bovarnick and her associates were forced to look for some more sensitive indicator of rickettsial well-being as a guide in approaching still closer to the goal of in vitro rickettsial growth. They chose protein synthesis because it is essential to growth and because very low levels of protein incorporation may be detected by the uptake of radioactive-labeled amino acids (Bovarnick *et al.*, 1959; Bovarnick and Schneider, 1960*a*). This work has already been discussed in the section on metabolic pathways, but it will be considered here from a different point of view— namely, the factors necessary for optimal rates of amino acid incorporation and their relation to the factors required for preservation of other rickettsial activities.

Since Hopps *et al.* (1956) had already failed to detect glutamate incorporation in high concentrations of rickettsiae suspended in simple media such as described in Diagram III-1, they immediately started with lower cell densities and a much more complex medium containing all the naturally occurring amino acids, together with asparagine, glutamine, and glutathione, most of the B vitamins, ribonucleosides and deoxyribonucleosides, DPN, Co A, diphosphothiamin, TPN, and the triphosphates of adenosine, guanosine, cytidine, and uridine. These constituents were contained in a high potassium-ion medium buffered at pH 7 with phosphate. Also present were bovine serum albumin and a soluble protein fraction derived from chick-embryo yolk sac. This medium was varied by omission of some constituents and the addition of still others.

Table III-3 compares the factors affecting maintenance of infectivity with those required for the occurrence of in vitro uptake of amino acids. As already pointed out, incorporation occurred only in an environment much more complex than that necessary for maximal stability of infectivity, toxin, and hemolysin. Optimum incorporation of glycine required the presence of all naturally occurring amino acids, and the omission of even a single amino acid—serine, threonine, or valine—significantly depressed the uptake. Either ATP or ADP was required, ATP being more effective, and the other ribonucleotides were also needed for prolonged uptake. Magnesium ion was essential for incorporation of

TABLE III-3

COMPARISON OF FACTORS NECESSARY FOR PRESERVATION OF INFECTIVITY AND OF ABILITY TO INCORPORATE AMINO ACIDS IN *R. prowazeki*

FACTOR	ESSENTIAL FOR	
	Infectivity	Incorporation
Yolk-sac protein..............	+	+
High K^+, low Na^+............	+	+
DPN.......................	+	+
Coenzyme A.................	+	+
Glutathione.................	+	+
Glutamine..................	+	+
Serine......................	0	+
Threonine...................	0	+
Valine......................	0	+
Adenosine triphosphate........	0*	+
Adenosine diphosphate........	0	+
Adenosine monophosphate......	0	+
Other ribonucleotide mono- and triphosphates..............	0	+
Mg^{++}......................	0	+
Mn^{++}......................	0	+

* ATP is not required for preservation of infectivity when glutamine is present.

both glycine and methionine, while manganous ion was stimulatory. None of these substances had any effect on infectivity under the conditions of in vitro incorporation. Since infective rickettsiae must have the ability to synthesize protein, we must assume that they may lose the ability to make protein in vitro and yet be able to infect cells and to resume protein synthesis intracellularly.

RICKETTSIAL METABOLISM AND THE PATHOGENESIS
OF RICKETTSIAL DISEASES

Although one of the prime objectives of biochemical investigations on infectious agents has long been the explanation of the pathogenesis of diseases caused by these agents in chemical terms, progress has been slow, and clear-cut success has been achieved in only a limited number of infectious diseases (see Braun, 1960). While it cannot be said that the pathogenesis of the rickettsioses can now be completely explained by the results of the metabolic investigations just described, it can be stated with certainty that the known metabolic properties of rickettsiae are closely related to their invasiveness and pathogenicity and that hopes for eventual satisfactory biochemical explanation are very good (see reviews by Cohn, 1960; Weiss, 1960).

In man, the pathology of epidemic typhus and Rocky Mountain spotted fever has been most thoroughly studied. In both diseases, the rickettsiae multiply chiefly within the endothelial cells lining the small blood vessels, and the major symptoms of the two diseases can be largely accounted for in terms of vascular damage resulting from the growth of the rickettsiae in these cells. Let us see how what we have learned about the metabolic behavior of rickettsiae can illuminate this bare statement of the central pathology of rickettsial diseases.

Penetration of the Host Cell

Cohn *et al.* (1959) studied the penetration of *R. tsutsugamushi*, the agent of scrub typhus, into mammalian cells in vitro. The rickettsiae were purified from yolk sac, and mouse lymphocytoblasts were grown in a horse serum–beef embryo extract medium. Standard numbers of rickettsiae and mouse cells were mixed in roller tubes for different periods, and then

71

the cells were scored for intracellular rickettsiae by direct microscopic examination.

When rickettsiae and cells were suspended in the serum-embryo extract medium, almost all the mouse cells contained one or more organisms within an hour at 37° C. Inactivation of the rickettsiae by heat, ultraviolet light, or formalin reduced penetration to almost zero, indicating that the rickettsiae play an active role in invasion of the host cell and are not passively ingested by phagocytosis. Killing the mouse cells also reduced penetration to a very low level. The act of penetration showed a dependency on temperature such as would be expected for an active metabolic process. When a balanced salt solution was substituted for the complete medium, penetration dropped off by 50 per cent. However, the effect of the serum and embryo extract could be completely reproduced by adding 1 per cent serum albumin to the balanced salt solution, suggesting strongly that the superiority of the complete medium over the balanced salt solution rested entirely in the stability-promoting effect of protein on rickettsiae already described in the preceding section. Divalent cations were also required for optimum penetration. In this respect the requirements for penetration resemble those for amino acid incorporation more than those for preservation of infectivity.

Next, compounds known to be involved in rickettsial metabolism were added to mouse cells and rickettsiae suspended in balanced salt solution. Of a large number tested, only L-glutamate, L-glutamine, and a mixture of α-ketoglutarate and L-aspartate were effective. Each raised the extent of penetration to that found in complete medium. Since glutamine gives rise to glutamate by deamination and α-ketoglutarate and aspartate form glutamate by transamination, all these effects may be ascribed to the availability of glutamate during penetration. Of many other substances tested, only DPN definitely fostered penetration, and its effect was less than that of glutamate. The action of glutamate on the penetration process appeared to be as an energy source for oxidative phosphorylation. Its effect was temperature-dependent and was blocked by the oxidative inhibitors cyanide, azide, and arsenite and by the decoupling agent dinitrophenol. However, added ATP was ineffective, suggesting that endogenously generated ATP is essential for invasion.

It is not yet clear whether the various factors shown to be essential for penetration act merely by maintaining the viability of the rickettsiae or whether they play some more specific role in the process. In any event, the experiments of Cohn *et al.* (1959) demonstrate that penetration of the host cell by rickettsiae is an active process carried out by metabolically competent organisms.

Gilford and Price (1955) have reported that DPN and Co A favor the absorption of spotted fever rickettsiae to guinea-pig tunica, a reaction they believe related to the virulence of the organism.

Rickettsial Toxin

Two properties of rickettsiae which immediately come to mind in attempting to explain how rickettsiae damage host cells and produce the symptoms of disease are their rapid, almost immediate, toxicity for mice and their ability to hemolyze rabbit and sheep blood. Shortly after Cox first cultivated rickettsiae in chick-embryo yolk sac, Gildemeister and Haagen (1940) reported that mice died only a few hours after injection of yolk-sac emulsions rich in murine typhus rickettsiae. Similar toxic activity was subsequently found in rickettsiae of epidemic typhus, scrub typhus, and spotted fever. Toxicity for mice is closely associated with viable organisms and is neutralized by specific antiserum. However, a number of observations indicate that multiplication is not required for toxicity: toxic symptoms are evident within 30 minutes of inoculation; they occur in mice inoculated with rickettsiae which do not infect these animals; the toxicity is not prevented by antirickettsial drugs; and, as has already been mentioned, infectivity may be reduced 4–5 logs by suitable exposure to ultraviolet radiation without appreciably lowering the toxicity. The mechanism of rickettsial toxicity has been studied by a number of workers (see especially Clarke and Fox, 1948; Paterson *et al.*, 1954; Neva and Snyder, 1955; Wattenberg *et al.*, 1955; Greisman and Wisseman, 1958). Their general conclusion was that administration of large numbers of viable rickettsiae produced direct injury to cells, particularly those of the vascular epithelium, leading to a loss of capillary permeability and subsequent leakage of plasma into the tissues. Blood volume decreased to a point where the blood pressure could not be maintained, blood pressure fell abruptly, and the animal died. It is generally assumed that many of the vascular disturbances seen in experimental and clinical rickettsial infections have a similar basis.

The requirements for preservation of toxicity in vitro have already been described. They are essentially the same as those found for penetration of host cells—maintenance of a high level of oxidative phosphorylation. This could mean that rickettsiae must actively invade the endothelial cells of the vascular bed in order to exert their toxic effect. However, ultraviolet light appears to prevent penetration but not toxicity. This apparent contradiction can be resolved by assuming that the toxic action of rickettsiae results from an enzymic attack on the surface of the host cell by particles which have absorbed but not necessarily penetrated.

Rickettsial Hemolysin

Clarke and Fox (1948) found that typhus rickettsiae slowly hemolyzed rabbit and sheep erythrocytes but not the erythrocytes of a number of other animals, including mice and men. As we have seen, this hemolytic activity is closely linked to infectivity, toxicity, and respiration, but its exact relation to the pathology of rickettsial diseases is unknown. In severe rickettsial toxemias of rabbits, massive in vitro hemolysis was sometimes observed (Paterson *et al.*, 1954), but this was never seen with other experimental animals. There has been speculation that hemolysis is, in some manner, an in vitro expression of the same property of rickettsiae as that which produces toxicity in vivo.

Snyder *et al.* (1954) found that the hemolytic activity of typhus rickettsiae against rabbit red cells was dependent on the presence of glutamate and magnesium ion and was inhibited by cyanide and other metabolic inhibitors. Tetracyclines interfered with hemolysis, but chloramphenicol did not. Bovarnick and Schneider (1960*b*), in a further study of the metabolic basis of rickettsial hemolysis, concluded that ATP is always essential for this activity. In metabolically intact organisms, this ATP is generated by the oxidation of glutamate. However, metabolically damaged rickettsiae can still hemolyze rabbit cells if they are furnished with exogenous ATP.

Reversible Variation in Virulence of Spotted Fever Rickettsiae

Price (1953*a, b*, 1954) and Gilford and Price (1955) have made extensive and important studies on the variation in virulence of *R. rickettsii* in the field and in the laboratory. Among the many factors affecting the virulence of this agent is its metabolic state. Price and Gilford started with the observation of Spencer and Parker (1930) that if ticks infected with a virulent strain of *R. rickettsii* were refrigerated for several months, the rickettsiae were no longer virulent for the guinea pig, although they infected the animals and immunized them against virulent strains. They also retained their original infectivity for chick embryos. When the ticks had a blood meal or were held at 37° C. for 2 days, virulence for guinea pigs was restored. A single yolk-sac passage served the same purpose.

Gilford and Price (1955) reproduced all important aspects of this phenomenon in vitro. When yolk-sac suspensions of guinea-pig–virulent rickettsiae were incubated at 25° C. for 60 hours, infectivity for both guinea pigs and chick embryos was lost. However, when *p*AB was present, only guinea-pig virulence was lost; chick-embryo virulence was retained, and the resulting population resembled that found in refrigerated ticks. If DPN, Co A, or *p*-hydroxybenzoic acid were also added, virulence for both hosts was retained. Avirulent rickettsiae from ticks or from incubation of virulent egg seed with *p*AB were restored to the virulent state by incubation with DPN or Co A. There is a remarkable parallel between the loss and restoration of virulence for the guinea pig and the reversible inactivation of typhus rickettsiae. However, spotted fever rickettsiae retain chick-embryo virulence under conditions that inactivate this property in typhus rickettsiae.

Virulent and avirulent *R. rickettsii* strains exhibited the same infective dose for chick embryos and produced the same concentrations of toxin and hemolysin in this host (Price, 1953*b*). They had the same nucleic acid content and equal ability to oxidize glutamate and Krebs cycle intermediates. Despite these similarities, the virulent strains multiplied in the guinea pig to a far greater extent than did the avirulent ones and killed 25–50 per cent of them, while the avirulent strains killed none. Obviously, there are still unrecognized factors in the pathogenesis of experimental spotted fever in the guinea pig.

Price (1954) has observed that when infected ticks molt, there is a dramatic decrease in the virulence of *R. rickettsii* for guinea pigs, presumably through some direct or indirect action of the molting hormone. Here again is an almost untouched area of biochemical investigation.

The General Metabolic Pattern of Rickettsiae

Some Possible Reasons for Their Restriction to Intracellular Habitats

Before attempting to answer for rickettsiae the crucial question posed in chapter i—why they grow so well within suitable host cells and so poorly outside them—let us bring together and summarize what we have learned about rickettsial biochemistry. In morphology and chemical composition the rickettsiae are indistinguishable from small bacteria, but they exhibit many metabolic peculiarities that probably stem from long adaptation to intracellular life.

Since they have no demonstrable action on glucose and glucose phosphates, these organisms are without a functional Embden-Meyerhof glycolytic cycle. It is barely conceivable that they are impermeable to glucose, but it is far more likely that they have lost the ability to synthesize one or more enzymes of the glycolytic cycle. A search for persisting "vestigial" individual enzyme components of the Embden-Meyerhof scheme would be very interesting. It seems logical to assume that the ancestors of rickettsiae possessed functional glycolytic cycles because the glycolytic enzymes are among the most widely distributed in nature and are generally assumed to have been a part of the enzymic equipment of our common primordial forebear. Also, there is a low but definite utilization of pyruvate in rickettsiae, which suggests that they once possessed enzymes for the formation of pyruvate from glucose. It may be pertinent to note that the rickettsia-like agent isolated from ticks by Suitor and Weiss (1961) oxidizes both glucose and glutamate.

Micro-organisms which do not glycolyze glucose to pyruvate exhibit some other major pathway of energy metabolism (see Gunsalus *et al.*, 1955). Many pseudomonads and heterofermentative lactobacilli have evolved non-glycolytic methods for the utilization of glucose, while the proteolytic clostridia hydrolyze protein and gain metabolic energy by oxidizing the liberated amino acids. Rickettsiae have solved their energy problem by oxidizing glutamate via the Krebs cycle. No obvious energetic advantage is gained by injecting fuel into the Krebs cycle furnace at the α-ketoglutarate step rather than at the citrate step, as is customary in most organisms. Glutamic dehydrogenase—the enzyme for oxidation of glutamate to α-ketoglutarate—is almost universally present in cells, but it usually functions in the reverse direction as a pathway for formation of glutamate from ammonia by the Krebs cycle. It appears as if, at some time in the evolutionary past of rickettsiae, for reasons which cannot even be guessed at, glucose and the glycolytic cycle were discarded as an energy-yielding mechanism and replaced by the already existing glutamate-glutamic dehydrogenase pathway. Bovarnick and Allen (1957*b*) observed that the low level of free glutamate in serum effectively reactivated rickettsiae after starvation at 36° C., and from this we may conclude that there is enough glutamate inside host cells to supply the energy requirements of rickettsiae.

Although the choice of glutamate as a chief energy source is a little unusual, the other known metabolic pathways in rickettsiae are entirely conventional. They oxidize glutamate in a Krebs tricarboxylic acid cycle, pass the liberated electrons on to molecular oxygen via the usual respiratory enzymes, convert the energy liberated by glutamate oxidation into the energy-rich phosphate bonds of ATP, and use them in the synthesis of protein, lipids, and, we may reasonably assume, other cell constituents as well.

The most unconventional thing about rickettsiae is their instability in simple salt solutions in which ordinary bacteria survive happily. This metabolic fragility appears to have two chief causes—an almost complete lack of endogenous energy sources and an inability to keep essential cofactors from leaking out of rickettsial cells. Most micro-organisms, including the malarial parasites, have considerable stores of endogenous substrates which they slowly oxidize for long periods of time when they are deprived of their usual energy sources, but rickettsiae have no such reserves and show no oxygen uptake at all when not supplied with an oxidizable substrate. We have seen that, at 36° C. in the absence of glutamate, ATP levels in rickettsiae fall rapidly, and infectivity, toxicity, hemolytic activity and oxidative capacity are concurrently lost (Bovarnick and Allen, 1957*b*). When glutamate is added to the inactivated rickettsiae, infectivity is never regained, indicating that some vital property of the organism is irreversibly damaged by brief substrate deprivation and the resultant drop in ATP. The requirement for the addition of all the amino acids and all the ribonucleotides for even minimal incorporation of one amino acid into rickettsial protein is further evidence for the almost complete lack of low-molecular-weight metabolites in rickettsiae (Bovarnick and Schneider, 1960*a*).

That DPN and Co A are lost from rickettsiae during in vitro incubation was first shown by Bovarnick and Allen (1954). Addition of DPN and Co A to rickettsiae inactivated by their loss restored infectivity and other associated properties, showing that these phosphorylated cofactors may also pass into these organisms. The penetration of ATP into rickettsial cells is demonstrated by its ability to prevent inactivation of rickettsiae at 36° C. (Bovarnick and Allen, 1957*b*). It must be something more than coincidence that these three phosphorylated compounds, all of which are not taken up intact by ordinary cells, are also required for pyruvate oxidation and extracellular survival in the malarial parasite. It seems both more probable and more profitable to assume that one of the mechanisms for successful adaptation to intracellular life is the acquisition of permeability to large, energy-rich cofactors and metabolites. However, as has been pointed out for malarial parasites, such an intracellular advantage becomes a lethal hazard extracellularly. In their relative impermeability to the Krebs cycle acids, the tricarboxylic acids in particular, the rickettsiae resemble most other cells and show that on occasion they, too, can exhibit selective permeability.

For reasons discussed at the beginning of this chapter, the nature of the metabolism of rickettsiae within host cells must be inferred from their behavior in vitro. The sensitivity of isolated rickettsiae to slight alterations in their environment, as well illustrated by the studies on amino acid incorporation, make such extrapolation very difficult. As conditions for the in vitro maintenance of rickettsiae have improved, the number of enzymic reactions known to occur in these organisms has steadily increased. One is forced to wonder just how much rickettsiae do for themselves inside their host cells.

In the absence of more complete information, the question of the basis for the obligate intracellular parasitism of rickettsiae must remain a topic of speculation. The most stimulating hypothesis is that these micro-organisms are bacteria which, in becoming adapted to intracellular life, have retained most of their major enzyme systems but have lost many mechanisms for buffering themselves against unfavorable changes in their environment, because such changes are no longer encountered in the constantly benign interior of the host cell. Thus, when they are placed in a highly artificial extracellular environment, they cannot adapt to such a radical change, their enzyme systems fail to function, and they die. It should be remembered that these agents are transmitted by arthropods and that ability to persist extracellularly probably would have little survival value in the evolutionary history of rickettsiae. It is interesting that the one agent that is readily transmitted without arthropod intervention, *C. burnetii* (see Table III-1), is much more stable extracellularly than any of the other rickettsiae.

This hypothesis suggests that rickettsiae depend on their host cells for a steady supply of glutamate and other substrates and cofactors and for a complex environment in which cellular integrity and function may be maintained. It suggests that artificial cultivation of rickettsial agents will eventually be possible.

REFERENCES

ALLEN, E. G., BOVARNICK, M. R., and SNYDER, J. C. 1954. J. Bact., **67**: 718–23.

ALLISON, A. C., and PERKINS, H. R. 1960. Nature, **188**:796–98.

BOVARNICK, M. R. 1956. J. Biol. Chem., **220**:353–61.

———. 1960. J. Bact., **80**:508–12.

BOVARNICK, M. R., and ALLEN, E. G. 1954. J. Gen. Physiol., **38**:169–79.

———. 1957a. J. Bact., **73**:56–62.

———. 1957b. *Ibid.*, **74**:637–45.

BOVARNICK, M. R., ALLEN, E. G., and PAGAN, G. 1955. J. Bact., **66**: 671–75.

BOVARNICK, M. R., and MILLER, J. C. 1950. J. Biol. Chem., **184**:661–76.

BOVARNICK, M. R., MILLER, J. C., and SNYDER, J. C. 1950. J. Bact., **59**: 509–22.

BOVARNICK, M. R., and SCHNEIDER, L. 1960a. J. Biol. Chem., **235**: 1727–31.

———. 1960b. J. Bact., **80**:344–54.

BOVARNICK, M. R., SCHNEIDER, L., and WALTER, H. 1959. Biochim. Biophys. Acta, **33**:414–22.

BOVARNICK, M. R., and SNYDER, J. C. 1949. J. Exper. Med., **89**:561–65.

BOZEMAN, F. E., HOPPS, H. E., DANAUSKAS, J. X., JACKSON, E. B., and SMADEL, J. E. 1956. J. Immunol., **76**:475–88.

BRAUN, W. (ed.). 1960. Biochemical aspects of microbial pathogenicity. Ann. N.Y. Acad. Sc., **88**:1021–1318.

CHANCE, B. 1952. Nature, **169**:215–21.

CLARKE, D. H., and Fox, J. P. 1948. J. Exper. Med., **88**:25–41.

COHEN, S. S. 1950. J. Immunol., **65**:475–83.

COHEN, S. S., and CHARGAFF, E. 1944. J. Biol. Chem., **154**:691–704.

COHN, Z. A. 1960. Bact. Rev., **24**:69–105.

COHN, Z. A., BOZEMAN, M., CAMPBELL, J. M., HUMPHRIES, J. W., and SAWYER, T. K. 1959. J. Exper. Med., **109**:271–92.

COHN, Z. A., HAHN, F. E., CEGLOWSKI, W., and BOZEMAN, F. M. 1958. Science, **127**:282–83.

Cox, H. R. 1938. U.S. Pub. Health Rept., **53**:2241–47.

FULTON, F., and BEGG, A. M. 1946. Great Britain M. Res. Council, Special Rept. Series, **255**:163–91.

GILDEMEISTER, E., and HAAGEN, E. 1940. Deutsch. m. Wchnschr., **66**: 878–80.

GILFORD, J. H., and PRICE, W. H. 1955. Proc. Nat. Acad. Sc. U.S., **41**: 870–73.

GREIFF, D., PINKERTON, H., and MORAGUES, V. 1944. J. Exper. Med., **80**: 561–74.

GREISMAN, S. E., and WISSEMAN, C. L., JR. 1958. J. Immunol., **81**:345–54.

GUNSALUS, I. C., HORECKER, B. L., and WOOD, W. A. 1955. Bact. Rev., **19**:79–128.

HAMILTON, H. L., PLOTZ, H., and SMADEL, J. E. 1945. Proc. Soc. Exper. Biol. Med., **58**:255–62.

HAYES, J. E., HAHN, F. E., COHN, Z. A., JACKSON, E. B., and SMADEL, J. E. 1957. Biochim. Biophys. Acta, **26**:570–76.

HOPPS, H. E., HAHN, F. E., WISSEMAN, C. L., JR., JACKSON, E. B., and SMADEL, J. E. 1956. J. Bact., **71**:708–16.

HOPPS, H. E., JACKSON, E. B., DANAUSKAS, J. X., and SMADEL, J. E. 1959. J. Immunol., **82**:161–71.

KARP, A. 1954. J. Bact., **67**:450–55.

KAUSCHE, G. A., and SHERIS, E. 1951. Ztschr. Hyg. Infektkrankh., **133**: 148–59.

KLEINSCHMIDT, W. J., HOLMES, D. H., and BEHRENS, O. K. 1956. Biochim. Biophys. Acta, **22**:277–83.

NEVA, F. A., and SNYDER, J. C. 1955. J. Infect. Dis., **97**:73–87.

ORMSBEE, R. A., PARKER, H., and PICKENS, E. G. 1955. J. Infect. Dis., **96**:162–67.

References

PARETSKY, D., DOWNS, C. M., CONSIGLI, R. A., and JOYCE, B. K. 1958. J. Infect. Dis., 103:6–11.

PATERSON, P. Y., WISSEMAN, C. L., JR., and SMADEL, J. E. 1954. J. Immunol., 72:12–23.

PLOTZ, H., SMADEL, J. E., ANDERSON, T. F., and CHAMBERS, L. A. 1943. J. Exper. Med., 77:355–58.

PRICE, W. H. 1953a. Science, 118:49–52.

———. 1953b. Am. J. Hyg., 58:248–68.

———. 1954. In: F. W. HARTMAN, F. L. HORSFALL, JR., and J. G. KIDD (eds.), The dynamics of viral and rickettsial infections. New York: Blakiston Co.

RIS, H., and FOX, J. P. 1949. J. Exper. Med., 89:681–86.

SALTON, M. R., 1960. In I. C. GUNSALUS and R. Y. STANIER (eds.), The bacteria. 1:97–152. New York: Academic Press.

SCHAECHTER, M., BOZEMAN, F. M., and SMADEL, J. E. 1957a. Virology, 3: 160–72.

SCHAECHTER, M., TOUSIMIS, A. J., COHN, Z. A., ROSEN, H., CAMPBELL, J., and HAHN, F. E. 1957b. J. Bact., 74:822–29.

SHEPARD, C. C., and TOPPING, N. H. 1947. J. Immunol., 55:97–102.

SMITH, J. D., and STOKER, M. G. P. 1951. Brit. J. Exper. Path., 32:433–41.

SNYDER, J. C., BOVARNICK, M. R., MILLER, J. C., and CHANG, R. S. 1954. J. Bact., 67:724–30.

SNYDER, J. C., and DAVIS, B. D. 1951. Fed. Proc., 10:419.

SPENCER, R. R., and PARKER, R. R. 1930. U.S. Pub. Health Service Hyg. Lab. Bull., 154:1–116.

STOKER, M. P. G., SMITH, K. M., and FISET, P. 1956. J. Gen. Microbiol., 15:632–35.

SUITOR, E. C., JR., and WEISS, E. 1961. J. Infect. Dis., 108:95–106.

TAKEMORI, N., and KITAOKA, M. 1952. Science, 116:710–11.

TOVARNICKIJ, V. I., KRONTOVSKAJA, M. K., and CEBURKINA, N. V. 1946. Nature, 158:912.

WATTENBERG, L. W., ELISBERG, B. L., WISSEMAN, C. L., JR., and SMADEL, J. E. 1955. J. Immunol., 74:147–57.

WEISS, E. 1960. In: W. BRAUN (ed.), Biochemical aspects of microbial pathogenicity. Ann. N.Y. Acad. Sc., 88:1287–97.

WISSEMAN, C. L., JR., HAHN, F. E., JACKSON, E. B., BOZEMAN, F. M., and SMADEL, J. E. 1952. J. Immunol., 68:251–64.

WISSEMAN, C. L., JR., JACKSON, E. B., HAHN, F. E., LEY, A. C., and SMADEL, J. E. 1951. J. Immunol., 67:123–36.

WISSIG, S. L., CARO, L. G., JACKSON, E. G., and SMADEL, J. E. 1956. Am. J. Path., 32:1117–33.

WYATT, G. R., and COHEN, S. S. 1952. Nature, 170:846–47.

ZINSSER, H. 1935. Rats, lice, and history. New York: Little, Brown & Co., Inc.

CHAPTER IV

The Psittacosis–Lymphogranuloma Venereum Group

The psittacosis–lymphogranuloma venereum group is composed of a large number of closely related obligate intracellular parasites which exhibit an almost identical morphology, multiply in host cells by means of a unique developmental cycle, and share a common antigen. They are differentiated one from the other by the presence of specific antigens, by their virulence for different natural and experimental hosts, and by the nature of the diseases they produce.

About thirty distinct members of the psittacosis–lymphogranuloma venereum group have been recognized (Meyer, 1958). They resemble one another so closely that results obtained with one or a few agents may frequently be applied to the entire group with considerable confidence. These agents[1]

---

[1] Members of this group are frequently referred to as "viruses," i.e., psittacosis virus, lymphogranuloma venereum virus, etc. However, it has been universally recognized since the first discovery of these agents that they do not conform to usual definitions of "virus," and more recent investigations clearly show that the use of the word "virus" in connection with the psittacosis-lymphogranuloma group is completely misleading and should be avoided. Therefore, the noncommittal term "agent" is used here. For the sake of brevity, the group will be referred to merely as the "psittacosis group."

In the following pages, the reader will be painfully impressed with the desirability of establishing a vernacular epithet for the psittacosis group of a verbal utility equal to "rickettsiae" and "plasmodia." Meyer (1953) has suggested that all members of the psittacosis group be included in the genus *Bedsonia*, named after Sir Samuel Bedson, who made the first comprehensive study of a member of this group. Among the numerous virtues of this suggestion is that it furnishes a euphonious group epithet, the "bedsoniae."

may be divided into three logical, but somewhat arbitrary, groups. The *avian agents* are primarily parasites of birds, but the more virulent strains may infect man and other mammals. The disease produced by parrot agents is called "psittacosis" (genus *Psittacus*), while the term "ornithosis" is frequently used to designate the disease produced by agents from non-psittacine birds. The *mammalian agents* are generally highly specific for their natural hosts and are not important sources of infection for man. The agents of meningopneumonitis, mouse pneumonitis, and feline pneumonitis are widely used laboratory strains, while other mammalian agents cause encephalitis, pneumonitis, and enzoötic abortion in cattle, sheep, and goats. These diseases of domestic herbivores are of widespread occurrence and cause economic losses of considerable magnitude. The *human agents* may be passed from person to person without the necessity of an animal reservoir. They include human pneumonitis strains closely related to, if not identical with, some psittacosis and ornithosis strains, the agent of trachoma, and the agent of lymphogranuloma venereum.

Agents of the psittacosis group do not have arthropod vectors but are transmitted directly from one vertebrate host to another. Psittacosis, ornithosis, and human pneumonitis are transmitted by droplet infection, trachoma by direct contact, and lymphogranuloma venereum by sexual intercourse.

Although certain psittacosis and ornithosis strains produce severe and often fatal pneumonitis in man, this is an exceptional host-parasite relationship in the psittacosis group. The relationship more truly characteristic of the group as a whole is one in which infection takes place in the young bird or mammal, with low mortality and little overt signs of disease. The host recovers, but the parasite is not destroyed. Instead, there follows a long-lasting inapparent infection in which the parasite remains in its host in a potentially virulent state and ready to be transmitted to new hosts under appropriate conditions.

There is good evidence that, in their multiplication within host cells, the psittacosis group micro-organisms synthesize their characteristic macromolecules with their own enzyme systems. However, unlike the plasmodia and the rickettsiae, these organisms give no signs of possessing energy-yielding enzyme systems (Moulder and Weiss, 1951a; Perrin, 1952; Allen and Bovarnick, 1957). Thus, in elucidating the metabolic properties of the psittacosis group, it has been necessary to rely heavily on inferences drawn from the behavior of the agents during intracellular multiplication and from the properties of isolated particles.

GROWTH AND MORPHOLOGY

Growth Cycle

Probably the most striking characteristic of the psittacosis group as a whole is the regular sequential appearance of structurally and functionally different particle types during multiplication of these agents in infected cells (see Bedson, 1959). A knowledge of this developmental cycle, or growth cycle, is the first requirement for an understanding of the basic nature of the group.

Soon after Lillie, Coles, and Levinthal almost simultaneously reported in 1930 that the agent of psittacosis appeared in the cells of infected animals as very small basophilic cytoplasmic particles, Bedson and his associates recognized all the main features of the growth cycle of the psittacosis agent by observing stained preparations of infected mouse tissues with the light microscope (Bedson and Bland, 1932, 1934; Bedson, 1933; Bland and Canti, 1935). Their work was confirmed and extended by Burnet and Rountree (1935) and Lazarus and Meyer (1939), who studied

86

psittacosis in the chorioallantoic ectoderm of the chick embryo; by Yanamura and Meyer (1941), who observed the growth of the psittacosis agent in tissue culture; and by Rake and Jones (1942), who showed that the agent of lymphogranuloma venereum undergoes a growth cycle in chick-embryo yolk sac entirely comparable to that of psittacosis. Later studies by Weiss (1949), Bedson and Gostling (1954), Swain (1955), and Officer and Brown (1960) added further details and showed that other members of the group exhibited growth cycles like those of the agents of psittacosis and lymphogranuloma venereum. Finally, the advent of the electron microscope and the ultramicrotome allowed the description of changes in particle morphology during the growth cycle to a much finer degree of resolution than could be obtained with the light microscope (Gaylord, 1954; Mitsui *et al.*, 1957, 1958; Tajima *et al.*, 1957; Higashi, 1959; Litwin, 1959, 1962; Litwin *et al.*, 1961).

From all this work reported over a period of almost thirty years, a simple and coherent sequence of events in the growth cycle of a member of the psittacosis group may be constructed. Unless specifically noted, this scheme is taken from the publications of Litwin (1959) and Litwin *et al.* (1961), which give detailed documentation. Infection is initiated by an elementary body, a particle about $0.3\,\mu$ in diameter and consisting of a limiting wall or membrane containing an electron-dense central body surrounded by a less dense peripheral material (Figs. IV-1, IV-2). The nature of the dense central body will be considered when the formation of the dense-centered particles during the growth cycle is discussed.

Absorption of psittacosis agents proceeds relatively slowly, maximum absorption in susceptible cell cultures being obtained in about 2 hours (Weiss and Huang, 1954; Officer and Brown, 1960). Once within the cell, the dense-centered

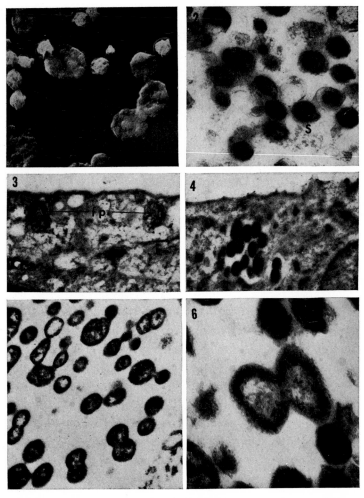

Figs. IV-1–IV-6.—Fig. 1: Electron micrograph of the agent of meningopneumonitis. Dried in air and shadowed with chromium. Reproduced from Moulder
(1962) by permission of the New York Academy of Sciences. 12,000×.

Figures IV-2–IV-11 are electron micrographs of thin sections of chorioallantoic
ectoderm or Chang's human liver cells infected with agents of the psittacosis group.
All are of osmium-fixed material except Fig. IV-3, which is of tissue fixed by the
freeze-dry technique of Gersh. Figures IV-3, -4, -5, -6, -8, -9, and -10 are reproduced
by courtesy of the indicated authors and the *Journal of Infectious Diseases.*

Fig. IV-2: The Borg strain of psittacosis in Chang's cells 45 hours after infection.
S =small dense-centered particle; L =large particle. Unpublished, courtesy Dr.
J. Litwin. 20,000×. Fig. IV-3: The agent of feline pneumonitis in the chorioallantoic ectoderm 1 hour after infection. fp =feline pneumonitis particles. From
Litwin (1959). 12,000×. Fig. IV-4: Psittacosis agent (strain 6BC) 12 hours after
infection of Chang's cells. From Litwin *et al.* (1961). 8,000×. Fig. IV-5: The
agent of meningopneumonitis in Chang's cells 20 hours after infection. From Litwin
et al. (1961). 8,000×. Fig. IV-6: The Borg strain of psittacosis in Chang's cells
30 hours after infection. From Litwin *et al.* (1961). 32,000×.

particle spends about 10 hours in an internal reorganization into a highly granular, coarse-meshed reticular form (Fig. IV-3) but never loses its morphologic integrity. We shall speculate on the chemical basis and significance of this change later in the chapter. The invading particle does not multiply until it is completely adjusted to its intracellular environment and has begun to form a space or vacuole around it. These large particles are normally the first evidence of infection to be seen with the light microscope and have been called "initial bodies," although such morphologic types persist throughout the growth cycle. From approximately 10 to 20 hours after infection, there occurs a slow but steady increase in particle number by fission of the large forms (Fig. IV-4). The organisms may be considered to be in their lag phase of growth, and, as with bacteria in the lag phase, it appears that a large amount of new agent material is synthesized with little division. This is the time when, particle for particle, the psittacosis group agents are most active in synthesizing their specific macromolecules and is the logical time to search for enzymic activity in these organisms. Unfortunately, the total particle number per host cell is still very low, and it is difficult to obtain substantial numbers of purified particles at this stage in the growth cycle. The large particles present during the lag period are definitely infective but much less so than the particles formed later in the infection.

At about 20 hours after infection of the host cell, the agent enters its logarithmic phase of multiplication. Total particle number increases logarithmically, division forms are numerous, and the internal structures of the log-phase particles are much less electron-dense than in the lag phase, suggesting that division is occurring at a faster rate than synthesis of internal material (Figs. IV-5, IV-6).

Some time around 20 hours after infection, at a time characteristic of each host-agent system, some of the large forms begin to differentiate into the small, highly infective, dense-centered particles (Fig. IV-7), which then cease to divide. Somewhat later, division of the large forms also ceases, the total particle count remains constant, but differentiation of large into small forms continues for a few hours (cf. Figs. IV-8 and IV-9). Finally, all activity halts, and the terminal population consists of a mixture of large and small particles, the relative proportions of which vary from about 30 to almost 100 per cent small, dense-centered forms, depending on the specific host-agent system involved. When the terminal population stage is reached, the host-cell cytoplasm is completely filled with infectious particles, and the cell ruptures to release the new generation to a brief extracellular existence and a search for new host cells. This phase of the growth cycle may be analogized to the stationary phase of the bacterial growth cycle. The dense-centered particle may be compared with the resting bacterial cell. It does not multiply, and it is more resistant to deleterious environmental factors than the lag- or log-phase particles. Its mode of formation is reminiscent of bacterial sporulation, but these forms have none of the properties characteristic of bacterial endospores. The rise in infectivity during the growth cycle closely parallels the appearance of the dense-centered particles, and, with the highly virulent strains of psittacosis, one chick-embryo infective dose is equivalent to one particle (Litwin *et al.*, 1961). The nature of the dense-centered body is unknown. It consists in large part of material other than DNA or RNA (Jenkin, 1960). The dense body probably represents some sort of generalized aggregation and condensation of the particle protoplasm which makes it incapable of division but renders it more resistant to the extracellular stresses it encounters in passing from one cell to another.

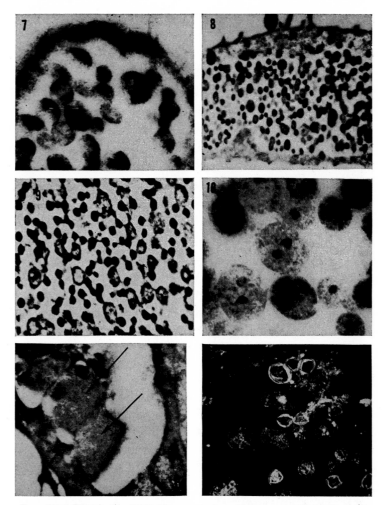

Figs. IV-7–IV-12.—Fig. IV-7: The agent of meningopneumonitis in the chorio-allantoic ectoderm at 20 hours. Unpublished, courtesy Dr. J. Litwin. 12,000×
Fig. IV-8: Psittacosis agent (strain 6BC) in Chang's cells at 25 hours. From Litwin et al. (1961). 4,000×. Fig. IV-9: Psittacosis agent (strain 6BC) in Chang's cells at 30 hours. From Litwin et al. (1961). 8,000×. Fig. IV-10: Like Fig. 9. Note multiple dense centers. From Litwin et al. (1961). 32,000×. Fig. IV-11: The agent of feline pneumonitis in the chorioallantoic ectoderm. The agent grew normally for 20 hours. Then 100,000 units penicillin per embryo were given via the yolk sac, and the membranes were fixed 5 hours later. Arrows indicate "penicillin forms." Unpublished, courtesy Dr. J. Litwin. 8,000×. Fig. IV-12: Electron micrograph of cell walls of the agent of meningopneumonitis. Air-dried and chromium-shadowed. From Jenkin (1960). Reproduced with the permission of the author and the *Journal of Bacteriology*. 9,000×.

Mechanism of Reproduction

Those who studied multiplication of the psittacosis group agents with the light microscope generally concluded that binary fission (division of a particle into two approximately equal daughter particles) was the principal mode of reproduction (Bedson and Bland, 1934; Bedson and Gostling, 1954; Swain, 1955; Officer and Brown, 1960). When thin sections of infected cells were examined with the electron microscope, particles almost certainly in process of binary fission were observed (Gaylord, 1954; Higashi, 1959; Litwin, 1959). In the chorioallantoic membrane infected with the agent of feline pneumonitis, binary fission was the only mode of multiplication seen by Litwin. However, both Gaylord and Higashi observed other forms of multiplication of the agent of meningopneumonitis growing in the chorioallantoic membrane and in Earle's L cells. They are budding (unequal division of a single particle) and multiple endosporulation (the formation of several small particles within a single large one). A fourth method of multiplication has been proposed by Tajima *et al.* (1957) from observations on an agent of bovine origin growing in mouse lung and meningopneumonitis growing on the chorioallantoic membrane. They conceive of new particles being formed by condensations within a viral matrix.

Litwin *et al.* (1961) made a comparative study of four agents (three strains of psittacosis and one of meningopneumonitis) growing in Chang's human liver cells and in the chorioallantoic membrane and were thus able to examine the possible reproductive mechanisms of the psittacosis group in a much broader context than had previously been possible. Structures which could be interpreted as particles being formed from a viral matrix were never observed in any of the eight host-agent systems studied, and it was concluded that such a reproductive mechanism could not be an important means of multiplication in the psittacosis group. Examination of many electron micrographs left little doubt that in all eight host-agent systems two particles frequently arose from the fission of one particle. Whether this division was equal (binary fission) or unequal (budding) is difficult to decide. Vagaries of sectioning angle could cause either mode of division to be mistaken for the other. Higashi (1959) has concluded that binary fission is most prominent in the early stages of the growth cycle, while budding is most important from about the twentieth hour onward. Litwin *et al.* (1961) did not observe such a shift in reproductive mechanism. They suggested that the fission mechanism in the psittacosis group is too rudimentary to be classified in either category; that is, division of a particle may occur at random in almost any plane, with resultant variation in the relative size of the two daughter particles.

The fission of a bacterium and a psittacosis agent are similar, in that no mitotic apparatus is visible at division. However, the psittacosis particles form no cross-wall between the two daughter cells before they separate (Figs. IV-5, IV-6), while the production of a cross-wall is characteristic of bacterial cell division (Bissett, 1956). Comparable observations are unfortunately not available for rickettsiae. The absence of a cross-wall is puzzling, since agents of the psittacosis group, like rickettsiae, possess cell walls that closely resemble those of bacteria (Jenkin, 1960).

Both Gaylord (1954) and Higashi (1959) interpreted the formation of multiple dense-centered particles such as those shown in Figure IV-10 in terms of a process of multiple endosporulation. However, Litwin *et al.* (1961) observed such particles only rarely in Chang's human liver cells and not at all in the chorioallantoic membrane, and only one particle with more than two dense centers (three) was ever seen.

These results do not support the idea that multiple endo-sporulation is a necessary and important mode of multiplication in the psittacosis group. The double dense-centered particles probably arise when the process of dense-center formation begins before the last division of a large particle has been completed.

Formation of Vesicles and Matrices

As soon as the initial body begins to divide, it commences to form a vacuole or vesicle, probably by enzymatic digestion of the surrounding cytoplasm. Note that in Figure IV-3 the single particles are still in intimate contact with the surrounding cytoplasm, while in Figure IV-4, the microcolony resulting from multiplication of an invading particle is already surrounded by a vesicle. The formation of the vesicle is an important part of the growth cycle of the psittacosis agent; for when the particles begin to multiply, they must have a space to expand into and a rich supply of nutrients, both of which are supplied by the vesicle and its fluid contents. Litwin (1959) has speculated that if the vesicle fluid could be reproduced in vitro, psittacosis group agents could multiply in it extracellularly.

When stained or unstained preparations of infected cells are examined with the light microscope, the vesicle appears to be surrounded by a wall or membrane (see Bland and Canti, 1935). However, no such limiting structure is seen with the electron microscope; the boundary of the vesicle is very irregular, with strands of cytoplasm extending from the periphery toward the center (Figs. IV-7, IV-8). It is possible that the membrane seen with the light microscope is the sharply demarcated phase difference between the structureless fluid of the vesicle and the highly organized unaltered cytoplasm.

The fluid or semifluid content of the vesicle was called

"matrix" by Bland and Canti (1935), who observed it in living infected cells. They noted that early in the growth cycle the matrix was very similar to the cytoplasm in viscosity and refractive index and that the viscosity lessened and the refractive index changed as the cycle progressed, until finally the particles could be clearly seen in rapid Brownian movement. These observations are nicely explained by assuming an enzymatic attack on the surrounding cytoplasm by the multiplying psittacosis agents. The matrix is of undetermined composition. Presumably it is as complex as cytoplasm itself. Psittacosis and ornithosis matrices are rich in RNA (Pollard *et al.*, 1960) while trachoma matrices are unique in their high content of a glycogen-like polysaccharide (Rice, 1936).

METABOLISM OF THE PSITTACOSIS GROUP

From the earliest times, many workers have felt that agents of the psittacosis group more closely resemble bacteria and rickettsiae than they do true viruses (see Bedson, 1959), and in recent years this conviction has been supported by a variety of experimental findings. It is now evident that these micro-organisms possess definite independent enzymic capabilities, although they appear to be even more limited than those of rickettsiae.

Preparation of Purified Suspensions

The necessity of working with agent preparations uncontaminated with host material is just as great in the psittacosis group as in rickettsiae. Some results have been obtained with preparations purified from chick-embryo yolk sac by essentially the same methods as those employed for rickettsiae (Moulder and Weiss, 1951a; Zahler and Moulder, 1953; Allen and Bovarnick, 1957), but most workers have started with infected allantoic fluid (see, for example, Gogolak and Ross, 1955; Allen and Bovarnick, 1957; Colón and Moulder,

1958). When growth of the psittacosis group agents is carried out in the allantoic cavity of the chick embryo under carefully controlled conditions, they are released from the infected entodermal cells lining the cavity without extensive concomitant release of host-cell debris, and concentrates of a satisfactory degree of purity may be obtained by several cycles of high- and low-speed centrifugation. Digestion with pancreatin or cobra venom may also be profitably employed at some stage in the purification (Allen and Bovarnick, 1957, 1960).

Criteria for freedom from host contaminants usually consist of the absence of host antigens in serological tests and the absence of particulate matter of recognizable host origin in electron micrographs. As with rickettsiae, the judicious use of normal host-cell controls is of critical importance in establishing that a given constituent or activity of a purified preparation is an intrinsic property of the agent and not of host-cell origin.

A complicating factor not encountered with rickettsiae springs from the presence of variable proportions of the two main morphologic types of particles in all purified preparations. Since we have just seen that there is good evidence that the enzymic activity and chemical comparison of the two types may not be the same, it is necessary to keep the complex nature of the particle populations in mind when interpreting results.

Chemical Composition

Agents of the psittacosis group are chemically complex organisms, with all the usual cell constituents. Of the common amino acids, only arginine and histidine are missing from the parasite protein (Gogolak and Ross, 1955; Jenkin, 1960). Jenkin has estimated that about 35 per cent of the dry weight of the meningopneumonitis agent is protein.

Micro-organisms of the psittacosis group have a large lipid content. Jenkin (1960) found phospholipid and neutral fat in meningopneumonitis, but no cholesterol. The phospholipid present in the 6BC strain of psittacosis has been positively identified as lecithin (Gogolak and Ross, 1955).

Both RNA and DNA are present (Zahler and Moulder, 1953; Ross and Gogolak, 1957*b;* Moulder, 1962). RNA readily leaks out of purified particles (Moulder, 1962), just as it does from rickettsiae and bacteria, and some workers have not

DIAGRAM IV-1

STRUCTURE OF MURAMIC ACID

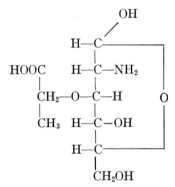

Muramic Acid

found it at all (Crocker, 1952; Gogolak and Ross, 1955). About 3.5 per cent of the dry weight of meningopneumonitis particles is DNA, while the RNA content varies from 2 to 7 per cent (Moulder, 1962). Gogolak and Ross (1955) and Ross and Gogolak (1957*b*) isolated the purine and pyrimidine bases from psittacosis (6BC strain). They found adenine, guanine, and cytosine in both, uracil in the RNA, and thymine in the DNA.

The agent of meningopneumonitis has about 2 per cent total carbohydrate, a third of which is hexosamine (Jenkin, 1960). Both meningopneumonitis (Jenkin, 1960) and mouse pneumonitis (Allison and Perkins, 1960) contain muramic acid, an amino sugar found only in bacteria, rickettsiae, and the blue-green algae (Diagram IV-1).

Nutritional Requirements for Multiplication

The work of MacCallum (1936) and of Yanamura and Meyer (1941) established beyond all reasonable doubt that members of the psittacosis group multiply only within living cells. The nature and extent of the nutritional demands of the psittacosis group agents have been greatly clarified by the results of Morgan and his associates. They found that the 6BC strain of psittacosis grows well in the L strain of mouse fibroblasts (Morgan and Bader, 1957). However, if the L cells were kept in a maintenance medium consisting of balanced salts and glucose for 2 days prior to infection, the 6BC agent infected such cells but was unable to multiply. If enriched medium was added at any time up to 4 days after infection of the depleted L cells, the psittacosis agent began to multiply at a normal rate. This furnished a sensitive system for studying the nutritional requirements for growth. A synthetic medium containing amino acids, B vitamins, glucose, and inorganic salts proved capable of stimulating propagation of the psittacosis agent in the depleted L cells. Systematic variation in the individual components of this medium then allowed the establishment of minimum nutritional requirements for psittacosis growth in L cells (Bader and Morgan, 1958, 1961). These requirements are listed in Table IV-1 and are compared with the requirements for growth of the L cells themselves, already established by Eagle (1955a, b). Glucose was also essential for psittacosis growth.

No amino acid or B vitamin not required for L-cell growth was essential for psittacosis multiplication. However, four amino acids and two vitamins necessary for multiplication of L cells were not required by the psittacosis agent. Of the four amino acids, arginine and histidine were not found in the agents of psittacosis strain 6BC (Gogolak and Ross, 1955) or meningopneumonitis (Jenkin, 1960), and the lack of any need for these amino acids probably reflects their complete or

TABLE IV-1

AMINO ACID AND B-VITAMIN REQUIREMENTS
FOR GROWTH OF L CELLS AND OF THE
AGENT OF PSITTACOSIS IN L CELLS

COMPOUND	REQUIRED FOR GROWTH OF	
	L Cells	Psittacosis Agent
Arginine*.............	+	0
Cysteine..............	+	+
Glutamine...........	+	0
Histidine............	+	0
Isoleucine...........	+	+
Leucine..............	+	+
Lysine...............	+	0
Methionine..........	+	+
Phenylalanine........	+	+
Threonine...........	+	+
Tryptophan..........	+	+
Tyrosine.............	+	+
Valine...............	+	+
Choline..............	+	±†
Folic acid...........	+	0
Nicotinamide.........	+	±
Pantothenic acid......	+	±
Pyridoxal............	+	±
Riboflavin...........	+	0
Thiamin.............	+	+

* Only L-amino acids were active.
† These B vitamins (±) required for maximum growth but not absolutely essential.

virtual absence from psittacosis protein. However, lysine is present in appreciable amounts in both the 6BC strain and the meningopneumonitis agent. The results of Jenkin (1960) show that it is a component of the bacteria-like cell wall, and it seemed likely that the members of the psittacosis group might, like bacteria, synthesize lysine via diaminopimelic acid (see Salton, 1960). Tests of this hypothesis with purified suspensions of the agent of meningopneumonitis showed that they could decarboxylate diaminopimelic acid to lysine, a reaction not occurring in higher animals (Moulder, 1962). Glutamine functions more as a coenzyme than as a constituent of protein, and the lack of a glutamine requirement for psittacosis growth is hard to assess. Its precursor, glutamic acid, is present in large amounts in psittacosis and meningopneumonitis protein. The lack of a folic acid requirement was to be expected from the demonstrated ability of the psittacosis group to synthesize this vitamin (Colón and Moulder, 1958; Colón, 1960, 1962). The absence of any need for riboflavin has special significance in light of the presence of an enzyme with the properties of a cytochrome *c* reductase in the meningopneumonitis agent (Allen and Bovarnick, 1957, 1960), for in higher organisms similar enzymes have riboflavin phosphate as their prosthetic groups.

Effect of Infection on the Metabolism of the Host Cell

Moulder and Weiss (1951*b*) compared the oxidative and glycolytic activity of normal chick-embryo yolk sac and yolk sac heavily infected with the agent of feline pneumonitis and found no difference. Zahler (1953) continued this comparison of normal and infected yolk sac by studying the effect of infection with feline pneumonitis on the concentration of phosphorus in the various fractions obtained in the usual Schneider-Schmidt-Thannhauser phosphorus partition (Volkin and Cohn, 1954): acid-soluble, lipid, RNA, DNA, and protein. There was no change in any of these fractions, but when he measured the uptake of inorganic phosphate into these fractions by using P^{32}-labeled phosphate, he found that infection greatly increased the rate of incorporation of inorganic phosphate into DNA and to a lesser but definite extent

100

into RNA. The rate of incorporation into the other fractions remained unchanged.

These experiments are difficult to interpret except in a very broad way. They show that infection with a member of the psittacosis group causes no change in the energy metabolism of the host cell but that it does alter the rates of nucleic acid synthesis. In general, most workers have felt that, within the limitation of present techniques, not much can be learned from studying the over-all metabolism of infected cells.

Energy Metabolism

The success of Bovarnick and Snyder in demonstrating the oxidation of glutamate by typhus rickettsiae (chap. iii) encouraged a similar search for oxidative activity in members of the psittacosis group (Moulder and Weiss, 1951a; Perrin, 1952; Allen and Bovarnick, 1957). However, all three groups agreed that the agents of feline pneumonitis, psittacosis, and meningopneumonitis not only did not oxidize glutamate but failed to oxidize other amino acids, pyruvate, and the acids of the tricarboxylic acid cycle. There was no oxidation when either molecular oxygen, DPN, or TPN was used as the oxidant (Allen and Bovarnick, 1957). Glucose was not phosphorylated in the presence of ATP and was not converted to lactate (Moulder and Weiss, 1951a).

The only oxidative reaction found in the psittacosis group is the oxidation of reduced DPN by cytochrome c in purified preparations of the agent of meningopneumonitis (Allen and Bovarnick, 1957, 1960). In other organisms, the reaction is catalyzed by a flavoprotein, cytochrome c reductase, and it may be tentatively assumed that a similar enzyme is responsible for the oxidation of reduced DPN in meningopneumonitis. This activity was proportional to the infectivity of the preparations, was lost when infectivity was destroyed by relatively mild inactivating agents, and resisted the action of trypsin and of lecithinases from *Clostridium per-fringins* toxin and cobra venom, which almost completely destroyed the cytochrome *c* reductase activity of normal host particle preparations. These observations lend strong support to the view that this activity is a true enzymic property of the meningopneumonitis particles. It seems doubtful that the meningopneumonitis cytochrome *c* reductase functions in the transport of electrons from substrates to molecular oxygen, for DPN-dehydrogenases and cytochrome oxidase—the enzymes on either side of cytochrome *c* reductase in the usual electron-transport chain—are absent. Allen and Bovarnick (1957) observed that other oxidants might replace cytochrome *c* and suggested that the reduction of some unknown oxidant might be the true function of the enzyme.

Although no hint of either aerobic or anaerobic energy-yielding reactions was found in the psittacosis group, the results of Moulder *et al.* (1953) showed that multiplication of the agent of feline pneumonitis in isolated yolk-sac fragments was highly dependent on the continued generation of energy-rich phosphate esters by the aerobic oxidations of the host cell. Anaerobiosis, azide, fluoride, and 2,4-dinitrophenol all inhibited oxidative phosphorylation and feline pneumonitis multiplication to the same degree. Other inhibitors, such as malonate and fluoracetate, which did not affect oxidative phosphorylation did not prevent growth of the agent.

These studies on energy metabolism may be interpreted in three different ways: (1) the energy-yielding enzyme systems of the psittacosis group agents are inactivated during purification; (2) the correct energy-yielding substrate has not been tested; and (3) the psittacosis group agents have no energy metabolism and depend on their hosts for a supply of high-energy metabolic intermediates such as ATP and acetyl-Co A. At present, not one of these hypotheses can be taken as proved, and not one can be discarded as completely untenable. We shall return to this problem at the end of the chapter.

Nucleic Acid Metabolism

Zahler and Moulder (1953) extended the investigations of Zahler (1953) on the nucleic acid metabolism of infected yolk sac by growing the agent of feline pneumonitis in yolk sacs labeled with radioactive inorganic phosphate and purifying the labeled virus. Although it is now obvious that their purified preparations were contaminated with host phospholipid (compare the analytical figures of Zahler and Moulder with the more recent ones of Jenkin, 1960), their results are still of significance, in that they showed that the specific activity of the RNA and DNA phosphorus was several times higher than that of any host phosphorus fraction at the time of isolation of the agent. This suggests that the feline pneumonitis nucleic acids were formed from simple precursors, including inorganic phosphate, and that, once formed, they were not in equilibrium with any host phosphate fraction. Pelc and Crocker (1961) used tritiated DNA precursors and a radioautographic technique to show that infection with psittacosis did not alter the rate of synthesis of nuclear DNA in HeLa cells and that psittacosis DNA and nuclear DNA were synthesized by independent pathways. All this evidence leads to the conclusion that members of the psittacosis group synthesize their own nucleic acids and depend on their host cells only for precursors of as yet unknown complexity. The hypothesis of Tanami *et al.* (1961) that there is a 10-hour lag between synthesis of agent DNA and its incorporation into particles is based on numerous errors of technique and assumption.

Since bacteria (reviewed by Mandelstam, 1960) and rickettsiae (chap. iii) frequently leak RNA under inimical conditions, it seemed likely that the RNA of the psittacosis group might be equally unstable. Rappaport and Moulder (see Moulder, 1962) investigated this possibility and found that both the RNA and the DNA of purified meningopneumonitis agent were stable at 0° C. and did not leak out of the particles. However, at 37° C., infectivity was rapidly lost, only the DNA was stable, and about half of the RNA leaked out of the particles in 12–18 hours and appeared in the supernatant as nucleosides. The great stability of the DNA is consonant with a role as the genetic material of the psittacosis group and is evidence for the presence of a functional nuclear body. The fact that only a portion of the meningopneumonitis RNA broke down at 37° C. suggests that the psittacosis group, like bacteria and other cells, contains more than one kind of RNA. This conclusion is also supported by the observation that 1 per cent serum albumin preserved the infectivity of purified meningopneumonitis almost without loss for 18 hours at 37° C. but was without effect on RNA leakage. It thus appears that the lost RNA is not vital and may be resynthesized when the depleted particle establishes itself within a host cell. In general, the occurrence of RNA is highly indicative of the presence of synthetic enzyme systems in the psittacosis group.

Effect of Antibacterial Agents

The multiplication of agents of the psittacosis group is inhibited by many chemotherapeutic agents effective against bacteria: the sulfonamides, penicillin, the tetracyclines, erythromycin, and chloramphenicol, to name only the most important ones (reviewed by Eaton, 1950; Hurst, 1953). Unless we make the unlikely assumption that each of these drugs modifies the metabolism of every type of susceptible cell in every potential host in such a way as to prevent agent multiplication without interfering with normal cell metabolism, we must assume that the antibacterial agents act on the

one common denominator of all possible host-agent systems
—the agent itself. In other words, we can scarcely escape the
conclusion that chemotherapeutic agents inhibit the growth
of members of the psittacosis group, just as they inhibit the
growth of bacteria, by interfering with enzyme systems in the
agents themselves. Thus the inhibitory effects of chemotherapeutic agents on the psittacosis group are guideposts pointing
the ways to regions of independent enzymic activity. However, these guideposts are helpful only if the traveler can
read the language in which their messages are written. To
put it more prosaically, one must work with inhibitors of
known mechanisms of action. The only chemotherapeutic
agents effective against the psittacosis group and with well-
understood modes of action are penicillin and the sulfonamides, and it is just these two agents that have been most
useful in the biochemical characterization of the psittacosis
group.

Biochemical Significance of the Susceptibility of the Psittacosis Group to Penicillin

Penicillin inhibits the growth of bacteria by interfering
with cell-wall synthesis (Hahn and Ciak, 1957; Lederberg,
1957; Park and Strominger, 1957). The specific reaction inhibited by penicillin appears to be the incorporation of a
muramic acid–containing peptide into the fabric of the cell
wall (Strominger *et al.*, 1959), as shown in Diagram IV-2.
Since these structures are unique to the bacteria and the
blue-green algae, the reason for the chemotherapeutic effec-
tiveness of penicillin is clearly revealed: it inhibits a reaction
in bacteria that has no counterpart in their hosts. Also explained is the well-known fact that penicillin kills only
multiplying bacteria. Cells multiplying in the presence of
penicillin are unable to form cell walls of normal strength and
rigidity and are consequently lysed in media of ordinary

osmotic properties. In media containing a non-penetrating solute to balance the internal osmotic pressure of the bacterial cell, new cells formed in the presence of penicillin may swell into uniformly spherical spheroplasts surrounded by a defective, non-rigid cell wall and an intact cell membrane. When penicillin is removed, some spheroplasts regain their normal morphology and resume multiplication. In the presence of penicillin, many bacteria are converted into stable L-forms, completely penicillin-resistant cells which produce progeny with defective cell walls and spherical shapes, even

DIAGRAM IV-2

SITE OF ACTION OF PENICILLIN

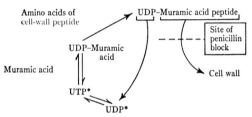

* UDP =uridine diphosphate; UTP =uridine triphosphate. This nucleotide is postulated to act as a catalytic carrier of the basic cell-wall unit, the muramic acid–peptide.

in the absence of the antibiotic (see Salton, 1960, and Mc-Quillen, 1960, for references).

The interaction between agents of the psittacosis group and penicillin may be explained by the same concepts as those developed from study of the action of penicillin on bacteria. In varying degree, all members of the group are susceptible to penicillin, the mammalian agents being generally more easily inhibited than the avian ones. Significant inhibition of the multiplication of the agent of feline pneumonitis in chick-embryo yolk sac may be obtained with as little as 10 units penicillin per egg, an initial concentration of about 0.2 unit per ml. (Moulder *et al.*, 1955). Since penicillin is rapidly destroyed in fertile eggs (Hamre and Rake, 1947;

Moulder *et al.*, 1956), this represents a susceptibility equal to that of bacteria generally classified as "penicillin-sensitive."

Weiss (1950) and Hurst *et al.* (1953) observed the formation of large, irregularly shaped, and vacuolated bodies when the agents of feline pneumonitis and lymphogranuloma venereum grew in the yolk sacs of embryos treated with penicillin. Tajima *et al.* (1959) and Litwin (personal communication) saw similar abnormal forms with the electron microscope (Fig. IV-11). These large, shapeless bodies produced in the presence of penicillin remained viable and resumed multiplication at a normal rate as soon as penicillin was removed by injection of penicillinase into the infected embryos (Moulder *et al.*, 1956). These observations are all in agreement with the conclusion that agents of the psittacosis group form structures analogous to bacterial spheroplasts inside their host cells, whose cytoplasm acts as an osmotically protective medium. It is unfortunately not possible to form psittacosis spheroplasts in vitro because multiplication is required for production of the penicillin effect.

Agents of the psittacosis group develop resistance to penicillin (Moulder *et al.*, 1955; Gordon *et al.*, 1957). They become resistant in a stepwise fashion comparable with the manner in which bacteria develop resistance (Demerec, 1948). Cross-neutralization tests revealed that the penicillin-resistant strain of feline pneumonitis was antigenically different from the parent strain (Moulder *et al.*, 1958). Since the neutralizing antigen is located in the cell wall (Jenkin *et al.*, 1961; Ross and Jenkin, 1962), this suggests that penicillin resistance in the psittacosis group develops through alteration in the cell wall. Moulder *et al.* (1958) and Woodroofe and Moulder (1960), under widely differing conditions of selection, obtained a number of closely related mutants of parent and penicillin-resistant feline pneumonitis agent that were all completely resistant to the multiplication-inhibiting

action of both penicillin and neutralizing antibody. These and other peculiar properties of this type of mutant suggested that a drastic alteration in cell wall structure had occurred. The non-neutralizing and penicillin-insensitive variants may be broadly analogous to the stable L-forms of bacteria.

Thus studies on the effect of penicillin on the psittacosis group led to the almost inevitable conclusion that these agents must possess cell walls like those of bacteria. Jenkin (1960) provided experimental confirmation of this suggestion by isolating the cell walls of the agent of meningopneumonitis by treating purified particles first with deoxycholate and then with trypsin. The structures so obtained had the size and shape of intact particles (cf. Figs. IV-1 and IV-12), contained only traces of nucleic acid, and were almost completely free of electron-dense internal material. In chemical properties, the meningopneumonitis cell walls resembled those of rickettsiae (chap. iii) and Gram-negative bacteria (Salton, 1960). They had no diaminopimelic acid but contained lysine instead. They also contained the amino sugar muramic acid, which, as already pointed out, has been found only in the cell walls of bacteria. Almost simultaneously, Allison and Perkins (1960) reported the presence of muramic acid in the agent of mouse pneumonitis, another member of the psittacosis group. It may therefore be assumed with reasonable confidence that agents of the psittacosis group contain enzymes which synthesize muramic acid and, in suitable combination with other precursors, incorporate it into their cell walls. It may be assumed with equal confidence that penicillin inhibits this incorporation and thus prevents multiplication.

Folic Acid Metabolism of the Psittacosis Group

The mode of action of sulfonamides on bacteria is so well understood that the susceptibility of some members of the psittacosis group to this class of chemotherapeutic agents

strongly implies that the psittacosis agents have an active folic acid metabolism. Sulfonamides inhibit the growth of bacteria by blocking the incorporation of pAB into the folic acid molecule (Diagram IV-3; Woods, 1940, 1960). Folic acid is an essential component of all living cells whose coenzyme forms are active in a variety of reactions involving enzymatic transfer of single-carbon units from one molecule to another (Huennekins *et al.*, 1958; Wright, 1960).

DIAGRAM IV-3*

BIOSYNTHESIS OF FOLIC ACID AND ITS INHIBITION BY
SULFONAMIDES AND FOLIC ACID ANALOGUES

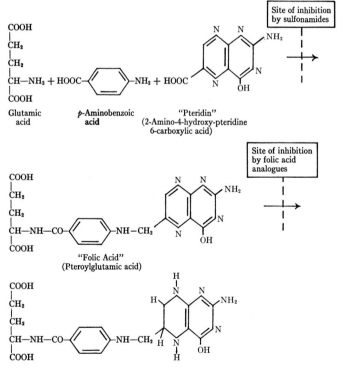

* Many details of this biosynthetic pathway are in doubt. The scheme is an approximation based on best available evidence.

Bacteria that make their own folic acid are sulfonamide-sensitive, while folic acid requirers are resistant because they do not carry out the reaction inhibited by the sulfonamides. All bacteria are inhibited by structural analogues of folic acid, such as aminopterin, because these inhibitors prevent the formation of the coenzyme form of folic acid (Diagram IV-3). Sulfonamide inhibition is competitively reversed by pAB and non-competitively by folic acid. Only folic acid reverses the action of its structural analogues.

Sulfadiazine is the sulfonamide of choice for treatment of both experimental and clinical infections with members of the psittacosis group. However, of the well-characterized members of the group, only the agents of lymphogranuloma venereum, trachoma, mouse pneumonitis, and a single strain of psittacosis virus (strain 6BC) are sulfadiazine-sensitive (see Eaton, 1950; Hurst, 1953). All the others are completely resistant to the largest doses of sulfonamides that can be administered. The susceptible members of the group quickly produce resistant mutants during multiplication in the presence of sulfadiazine (Golub, 1948; Loosli *et al.*, 1955). Both sulfonamide-sensitive and sulfonamide-resistant agents are inhibited by folic acid analogues, such as aminopterin and amethopterin (Morgan, 1952; Colón, 1959). These findings have important implications when interpreted in terms of the Woods-Fildes theory of the mechanism of action of the sulfonamides (Woods, 1952). Animals cannot synthesize folic acid from pAB and its other components and are therefore sulfonamide-insensitive. If sulfadiazine inhibits the growth of a micro-organism of the psittacosis group in an infected host cell, it must be assumed that the agent itself is capable of synthesizing folic acid from simple components and that this synthesis is necessary for its reproduction. It may be further supposed that the sulfonamide-resistant members of the psittacosis group have lost the ability to make the vitamin and now require an exogenous supply.

Further analysis of the effect of sulfadiazine on the multiplication of the psittacosis group gave solid support to these suggestions. Findlay's (1940) observation that pAB reverses inhibition of multiplication of the lymphogranuloma agent by sulfonamides was confirmed by the more extensive work of Morgan (1948, 1952) with the 6BC strain of psittacosis and by Huang and Eaton (1949) with lymphogranuloma venereum and mouse pneumonitis. pAB was a competitive antagonist of sulfadiazine, while pteroylglutamic acid and leucovorin reversed the action of sulfadiazine non-competitively. The ratio of pAB to sulfadiazine required for 50 per cent reversal was comparable to that found with bacteria.

With this strong indication that the psittacosis group has a folic acid metabolism equivalent to that of bacteria, Colón and Moulder(1958) sought direct evidence for the presence of folic acid in purified preparations of psittacosis group micro-organisms. Analysis of purified suspensions of the agents of feline pneumonitis, meningopneumonitis, mouse pneumonitis, and psittacosis (6BC) by microbiological assay and by paper chromatography-bioautography showed a relatively constant free folic acid content of a magnitude comparable with that of bacteria. Since the folic acid concentration in the purified preparation was very low, as it is in all cells, the usual criteria for freedom from host contamination were entirely inadequate to decide whether or not this folic acid was an intrinsic component of the micro-organisms or merely an adventitious host contaminant. Therefore, evidence was sought that would be independent of the degree of purity of the preparations. The folic acid in these purified suspensions was closely associated with the infectious particles and could not be separated from them without loss of infectivity. In addition, the forms of folic acid found in the

agent preparations did not occur in the normal host tissue—
the chorioallantoic membrane—or in allantoic fluid. However, the most convincing reasons for believing that folic acid
is a true constituent of members of the psittacosis group was
derived from observing that the kind and amount of folic
acid in a purified agent suspension was different for each of
the four agents studied. Table IV-2 shows that quantitative

TABLE IV-2

FOLIC ACID COMPOSITION OF AGENTS OF PSITTACOSIS GROUP

MEASUREMENT	AGENT ANALYZED*			
	Feline Pneumonitis	Meningo-pneumonitis	Mouse Pneumonitis	Psittacosis (6BC)
Susceptibility to sulfadiazine.	0	0	+	+
μg "Folic acid" per gram nitrogen as assayed with				
Lactobacillus casei†	27	21	47	14
Pediococcus cerevisiae‡ . . .	24	14	16	3
Relative concentration of active components with Rf's§ of				
0.65	+ +	+ + + +	+ +	+ + + +
0.55	+ +	+ + +	+ +	+ + +
0.40	+ + +	+	+ + +	+
0.20	+	+	+	+

    * Six to nine preparations of each agent were analyzed.
    † This organism responds to compounds of a complexity as great as, or greater than, pteroylglutamic acid.
    ‡ This organism responds only to compounds with a reduced pteridine nucleus, such as leucovorin.
    § Rf in isoamyl alcohol–5 per cent dibasic sodium phosphate, pH 9; 25° C.; ascending technique.

microbiological assay with two assay organisms and paper
chromatography, followed by bioautographic visualization of
active components, yielded a unique combination of results
for each of the four agents.

    There are no clear-cut analytical differences between
sulfonamide-sensitive and sulfonamide-resistant agents. A
high leucovorin–pteroylglutamic acid ratio was associated
with resistance, but the chromatogram of each naturally
resistant organism resembled one of the sensitive ones more

than the other resistant organism. Analysis of an artificially resistant strain of psittacosis 6BC (Golub, 1948) yielded results intermediate between the original resistant and sensitive pairs (Colón, 1959).

The conclusion that folic acid is an essential constituent of members of the psittacosis group led immediately to the hypothesis that these organisms must contain enzymes requiring and synthesizing folic acid coenzymes. Colón (1960, 1962) presented evidence for the existence of folic acid–synthesizing enzymes in the agents of mouse pneumonitis and meningopneumonitis. He described two different mechanisms whereby folic acid was formed in purified suspensions of these agents. If suspensions were incubated at 37° C. in the absence of any added substrate, there was an endogenous formation of material active for both *Lactobacillus casei* and *Pediococcus cerevisiae*. The sulfonamide-sensitive mouse pneumonitis agent exhibited a much higher rate of endogenous folic acid synthesis than did the sulfonamide-resistant agent of meningopneumonitis. Moreover, endogenous folic acid formation in mouse pneumonitis was inhibited by sulfadiazine, while the drug had no effect on the low endogenous rate in meningopneumonitis, thus providing an enzymic explanation for the differential drug susceptibility of the two organisms. Normal host-tissue preparations showed no endogenous folic acid formation, and the new folic acid synthesized in each purified suspension was chromatographically characteristic of that particular agent.

Conjugases—enzymes which break down polyglutamyl derivatives of folic acid to forms active in cell metabolism—were present in both purified agent suspensions and in normal chorioallantoic membrane preparations (Colón, 1960, 1962). However, the agent enzymes could easily be distinguished from the host enzymes by differences in substrate specificity, pH optimum, and cofactor requirements. There was also an interesting difference in substrate specificity between mouse pneumonitis and meningopneumonitis. Both could release active folic acid from extracts of purified agent suspensions, *Escherichia coli*, and baker's yeast, but only the sulfonamide-resistant meningopneumonitis agent could form folic acid from extracts of chorioallantoic membrane, allantoic fluid, and chicken serum. Since conjugase activity is not inhibited by sulfonamides, this would give the meningopneumonitis agent a sulfonamide-resistant source of folic acid but make the mouse pneumonitis agent completely dependent on the sulfonamide-sensitive endogenous pathway.

These observations are summarized in Diagram IV-4. All that remains is to show that enzymes with folic acid coenzymes are present and functioning in the psittacosis group micro-organisms.

BIOCHEMICAL PROPERTIES OF THE PSITTACOSIS GROUP AND PATHOGENESIS

Biochemical studies have so far contributed little to the understanding of the diseases produced by members of the psittacosis group. However, several important questions concerning the pathogenesis of these diseases may now be phrased in chemical terms. This is progress of a sort, for questions cannot be answered until they are asked.

Invasion

Considerable quantitative data on the efficiency with which organisms of the psittacosis group infect host cells have been obtained by counting the number of particles in suspensions of infective agents with the light microscope (Lazarus and Meyer, 1939; Gogolak, 1953; Manire and Smith, 1959; Smith and Manire, 1959) or the electron microscope (Crocker and Bennett, 1952; Crocker, 1954; Litwin, 1959, 1962; Jenkin, 1960; Litwin *et al.*, 1961) and inoculating the counted

114

suspensions into the yolk sacs of chick embryos for determination of their LD_{50} (50 per cent lethal dose). When terminal populations present at the end of the growth cycle were employed, the total particle/LD_{50} ratio varied from almost one for the 6BC and Borg strains of psittacosis (Litwin *et al.*, 1961) to a million for the agent of trachoma (Litwin, 1962). While infectivity in a single host by a single route of inoculation is only a limited measure of the invasiveness of an agent,

DIAGRAM IV-4

INTERRELATIONSHIPS OF DIFFERENT FORMS OF FOLIC ACID AND FOLIC
ACID PRECURSORS IN CELLS INFECTED WITH
PSITTACOSIS GROUP AGENTS

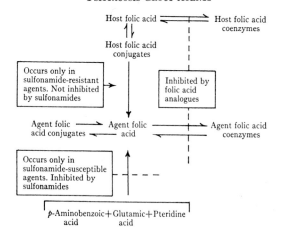

there is excellent correlation between the particle/LD_{50} ratio for yolk sac and host range and tissue tropism. Agents with particle/LD_{50} ratios near unity are invariably highly infectious for a variety of hosts and invade and grow in many different kinds of cells, while organisms with high ratios are restricted in host range and multiply in a limited number of tissues and cells.

The near-perfect efficiency of infection shown by the Borg and 6BC strains of psittacosis is indicative of a specific mode of invasion, for it is unlikely that a one-to-one ratio of total particles to infectious units would be attained via a passive and non-specific penetration of the host cell. Such a mechanism could involve specific complementary absorption sites on agent and host cell or active enzymic attack upon the host cell by the micro-organism or possibly a combination of both. We may assume that this postulated invasion mechanism would be absent or defective in inefficient agents, such as that of trachoma.

One definite piece of information bearing on the problem is that a site or structure intimately involved in the process of invasion is located in the cell walls of the psittacosis group agents. Jenkin *et al.* (1961) and Ross and Jenkin (1962) showed that neutralizing antibody—antibody which combines with the agent and makes it non-infective—may be absorbed specifically by isolated cell walls of meningopneumonitis agent. It should be possible to separate this "neutralizing antigen" from intact cell walls and to study it further.

Another phenomenon which should be of value in studying invasion mechanisms is the one hundred to one thousand fold drop in the particle/LD_{50} ratio that takes place between the fifteenth and twenty-fifth hours of the growth cycle (Litwin, 1959; Litwin *et al.*, 1961). There must be some definite chemical change accompanying this dramatic biological one. The proportion of dense-centered particles in the population increases several fold during this period, but Litwin *et al.* (1961) have shown that the sharp rise in infectivity precedes by about 5 hours the rise in dense-centered bodies.

Latency

As mentioned at the beginning of this chapter, a condition of latency is characteristic of natural infections with members of the psittacosis group. These agents persist for long periods of time in the tissues of man (Meyer and Eddie, 1951), mice (Bedson, 1938; Early and Morgan, 1946), and chick embryos (Davis and Vogel, 1949; Greenland, 1961) without obvious harm to these hosts, and the same situation probably exists in many other psittacosis group infections as well.

The mechanism of latency has been experimentally approached by Morgan and his associates in experiments already discussed in the section on nutritional requirements for growth. Morgan (1956) found that primary cultures of chick-embryo cells lost their capacity to support multiplication of the 6BC strain of psittacosis when maintained for 11–28 days in a simple inorganic salt solution. However, infection actually occurred under these conditions because the addition of beef extract to the starved cells up to 15 days after contact with the psittacosis agent resulted in active multiplication. Thus the agent remained for up to 2 weeks in a latent and undetectable form.

Morgan's group turned to mouse fibroblast (L cells) cultures for analysis of this nutritional effect because, although latent infections could be maintained for only 3 days in L cells, the system could be subjected to the more detailed nutritional study already described (Morgan and Bader, 1957; Bader and Morgan, 1958, 1961). Their results shown in Table IV-1 have already been discussed. It is sufficient for the purposes at hand to remind ourselves that (1) invasion of host cells is not dependent on their nutritional state, (2) multiplication does not occur when the host cell is deficient in certain amino acids and B vitamins, and (3) multiplication is initiated when the missing nutrients are supplied. Thus, as Morgan's group has suggested, latency may result from nutritional deficiencies in host cells, and recrudescences of frank disease may result when these deficiencies are corrected. One may rightly object that the cells of living intact animals are unlikely to reach the state of starvation achieved by maintaining isolated cells in balanced salt solution. However, it is now clearly evident that the absolute and relative concentrations of metabolites within cells are determined by a variety of complex regulatory mechanisms, and it seems entirely conceivable that the intracellular concentration of a metabolite essential for psittacosis growth might fall below the minimum required level under one set of conditions and rise above it under another, all in an adequately nourished host.

Although direct evidence is lacking and would be difficult to obtain with existing techniques, it seems likely that the infective agent invades the nutritionally deficient host cell with ease but is unable to undergo the extensive internal reorganization required for transformation of the invading particle into a vegetative multiplying one (see section on "Growth Cycle"). In other words, the stage in the growth cycle normally taking about 10 hours may be indefinitely prolonged in nutritionally deficient cells. Morgan and his associates probably found no infectivity in their experimental latent periods because of the drop in infectivity occurring soon after invasion and because the intracellular infectivity early in the growth cycle is destroyed by freezing and can be demonstrated only by immediate titration of fresh extracts (Litwin, 1959; Officer and Brown, 1960).

Litwin (1959) has described a second method for producing experimental latency. The chorioallantoic ectoderm was infected with the agent of feline pneumonitis. Then, 12–15 hours later, the particles present at this early stage in the growth cycle were inoculated onto other chorioallantoic membranes. The cycle was greatly delayed, and 90 hours elapsed before particles capable of initiating a normal growth cycle appeared. If this delayed cycle was interrupted at 50 hours and a third transfer of infectivity made, the cycle was again delayed, and fully infectious particles did not appear. In this manner, the agent of feline pneumonitis could be transferred indefinitely from one embryo to another without the appearance of normal infectious virus. However, no genotypic change occurred, for this "latent" agent always eventually produced normal progeny either on the chorioallantoic membrane or in the yolk sac. Litwin's results might also be explained by assuming that rapid transfer also indefinitely prolonged the early stages of the normal growth cycle.

It is therefore now possible to approach the fundamental biological problem of latency in the psittacosis group in terms of nutrition of the host cell and of alterations in the normal growth cycle of these organisms.

Toxin

The multiplication of an agent of the psittacosis group in the cytoplasm of its host cell appears to do little damage to the cell in areas not actually occupied by the multiplying particles. Although growth of these agents in cell cultures leads to eventual cell destruction (Weiss and Huang, 1954; Benedict and McFarland, 1958; Officer and Brown, 1960), cytopathic effects are rapid and severe only with such highly virulent strains as Borg, and chronic infections are readily established (Manire and Galasso, 1959; Officer and Brown, 1961). Cells in active mitosis may contain large inclusions, and one of the daughter cells may be normal in appearance and apparently uninfected (Officer and Brown, 1961). Thus direct damage to infected cells by multiplying particles does not seem sufficient to explain the pathogenicity and lethality of the agents of the psittacosis group for their intact animal hosts.

Under such circumstances it is customary to invoke the production of a toxin that is transported from the infected cell to especially susceptible distant sites, where it produces cell damage leading to pathology and death. Rake and Jones

(1944) and Manire and Meyer (1950) have shown that the psittacosis group forms a toxin closely associated with the infectious particles that is rapidly lethal for mice on intravenous injection. Multiplication is not essential for evocation of the toxic effect: the immunologic specificity of the toxin neutralization reaction is identical with, or very similar to, that of the infectivity neutralization reaction (Manire and Meyer, 1950); the toxic antigen is located in the cell wall, as is the neutralizing antigen (Ross and Jenkin, 1962; Manire, personal communication); and the toxic LD_{50} for mice is more than one million times the infectious LD_{50} dose (Manire and Smith, 1959). These observations suggest that the "toxin" of the psittacosis group is a reflection of the damage done to host cells during the act of invasion and that the toxin neutralization and infectivity neutralization reactions are titrating the same antigen, a substance or grouping on the cell wall that is intimately involved in invasion of cells. While this is a fascinating area for more work, it does not seem likely that the toxic effect demonstrated by the intravenous inoculation of mice with large numbers of infective particles plays an important role in the pathogenesis of natural infections with members of the psittacosis group.

This does not eliminate the possibility of the elaboration of other toxic substances, for several other soluble antigens of unknown toxicity are also produced during multiplication (Hilleman *et al.*, 1951; Gogolak and Ross, 1955; Benedict and O'Brien, 1958). Greenland (1961) has also obtained results with a mutant of penicillin-resistant feline pneumonitis that are most reasonably explained in terms of the existence of a lethal toxin whose synthesis or release is inhibited by penicillin.

However, it must be admitted that biochemical explanation of the damaging effects of micro-organisms of the psittacosis group on isolated cells and on intact hosts is entirely inadequate and that much work remains to be done.

Hemagglutinin

During their multiplication in host cells, micro-organisms of the psittacosis group produce a complex soluble antigen which specifically agglutinates mouse erythrocytes (Hilleman *et al.*, 1951; Gogolak, 1954; Gogolak and Ross, 1955). This hemagglutinin is a lecithin-DNA-protein complex similar in many respects to the hemagglutinin of the pox group of viruses (see chap. v). It is serologically related to a chemically similar antigen in the intact particles, but hemagglutinating activity cannot be demonstrated in intact or disrupted particles. How and why the psittacosis hemagglutinin is formed and what, if any, role it has in pathogenesis are completely unknown.

Summary

We have seen that some beginning has been made in understanding infections with organisms of the psittacosis group in terms of their known biochemical properties and behavior. It is painfully obvious that only a start has been made. Particularly lacking are biochemical data reflecting the great differences in biological behavior among agents of closely similar morphology. For example, small dense-centered particles of the Borg strain of psittacosis and the trachoma agent are indistinguishable in the electron microscope (Litwin, 1962; Litwin *et al.*, 1961), yet one can hardly imagine agents of more widely different properties. There must be corresponding differences in chemical composition and metabolic behavior if we were only wise enough and perceptive enough to see them.

SPECULATIONS ON THE BIOCHEMICAL BASIS OF
OBLIGATE INTRACELLULAR PARASITISM
IN THE PSITTACOSIS GROUP

All evidence points to the conclusion that organisms of the psittacosis group possess enzyme systems capable of synthesizing the macromolecules of protein and nucleic acid specific for each agent, as well as low-molecular-weight metabolites, such as folic acid, lysine, and muramic acid, that are not synthesized by their hosts. Although it is hard to assess the magnitude and level of the demand, they certainly depend on their hosts for supplies of many other small metabolites which they obtain by tapping their hosts' free metabolite pools or by digesting host cytoplasm. Whether the chemical complexity of this substrate demand is high enough to prevent its being met outside living cells either artificially or by natural intracellular fluids is impossible to determine at present.

The most obvious metabolic deficiency in these organisms is their apparent lack of any sort of energy metabolism. We have already suggested three possible interpretations: (1) the energy-yielding systems are inactivated during purification, (2) the correct energy-yielding substrate has not been tested, or (3) the psittacosis group depend on their hosts for supplies of such high-energy metabolites as ATP and other nucleotide triphosphates, acetyl–Co A, etc.

The first possibility seems unlikely because the psittacosis group agents are relatively stable in the cold. Purified suspensions with particle/LD_{50} ratios equal to those of the crude starting material may be obtained with relative ease, and yet they have no oxidative activity (Moulder, unpublished results). Highly purified preparations of meningopneumonitis agent are rapidly inactivated at 37° C., but most of this loss of infectivity may be prevented by the addition of calcium ion (Allen and Bovarnick, 1957) or serum albumin (Moulder, 1962). If we are to explain the lack of energy metabolism in the psittacosis group on the basis of enzyme inactivation during purification and testing, we must postulate that enzyme activity is lost more rapidly than infectivity, an assumption counter to all other experience.

The second explanation is difficult to refute because, no matter how many negative experiments are run, the next experiment with an untried potential substrate may be positive. However, it too seems unlikely, chiefly because Allen and Bovarnick (1957) have shown that the usual electron-transport systems are absent. Thus we should have to postulate the existence not only of an esoteric energy-yielding substrate but also of an equally esoteric pathway of electron transport.

This leaves us with the third explanation—that the psittacosis group micro-organisms are energy parasites. For example, they may synthesize their own DNA if supplied with the appropriate nucleotide triphosphates (see Davidson, 1960), their own protein if given activated amino acids (see Hoagland, 1960), and their own fatty acids if given acetyl–Co A, ATP, and reduced TPN (see Stumpf, 1960). Such ideas require the agents of the psittacosis group to be permeable to these energy-rich compounds, which are all highly polar and do not easily penetrate most cell membranes. However, we saw in chapters ii and iii that there is good evidence that ATP, DPN, Co A, etc., freely pass in and out of malarial parasites and rickettsiae. This evidence was obtained by showing that the addition of these compounds promoted survival and increased the rate of various enzyme reactions. It should be possible to apply these methods to the psittacosis group, and it is certainly possible to study directly the uptake of ATP, for example, with molecules suitably tagged with isotopic labels. If agents of the psittacosis group are found to be permeable to high-energy compounds and if energy-yielding reactions are not found upon further search, it will appear very probable that the psittacosis group organisms depend on their hosts to generate energy-rich intermediates for them. Such a dependency would be a sufficient explanation for the obligate intracellular parasitism of these organisms because it is most unlikely that an adequate concentration and variety of high-energy compounds will be found outside living, actively metabolizing cells.

REFERENCES

ALLEN, E. G., and BOVARNICK, M. R. 1957. J. Exper. Med., **105**:539–47.

———. 1960. Virology, **11**:737–52.

ALLISON, A. C., and PERKINS, H. R. 1960. Nature, **188**:796–98.

BADER, J. P., and MORGAN, H. R. 1958. J. Exper. Med., **108**:617–30.

———. 1961. *Ibid.*, **113**:271–81.

BEDSON, S. P. 1933. Brit. J. Exper. Path., **14**:267–77.

———. 1938. *Ibid.*, **19**:353–66.

———. 1959. J. Roy. Inst. Pub. Health Hyg., **22**:67–78.

BEDSON, S. P., and BLAND, J. O. W. 1932. Brit. J. Exper. Path., **13**:461–66.

———. 1934. *Ibid.*, **15**:243–47.

BEDSON, S. P., and GOSTLING, J. V. T. 1954. Brit. J. Exper. Path., **35**: 299–308.

BENEDICT, A. A., and McFARLAND, C. 1958. Nature, **181**:1742–43.

BENEDICT, A. A., and O'BRIEN, E. 1958. J. Immunol., **80**:94–99.

BISSETT, K. A. 1956. *In:* Bacterial anatomy: 6th symposium of the Society for General Microbiology, ed. E. T. C. SPOONER and B. A. D. STOCKER, pp. 1–18. Cambridge: Cambridge University Press.

BLAND, J. O. W., and CANTI, R. G. 1935. J. Path. Bact., **40**:231–41.

BURNET, F. M., and ROUNTREE, P. M. 1935. J. Path. Bact., **40**:471–81.

COLÓN, J. I. 1959. Doctoral dissertation, University of Chicago.

———. 1960. J. Bact., **79**:741–46.

———. 1962. Ann. N.Y. Acad. Sc., in press.

COLÓN, J. I., and MOULDER, J. W. 1958. J. Infect. Dis., **103**:109–19.

CROCKER, T. T. 1952. Fed. Proc., **11**:464–65.

———. 1954. J. Immunol., **73**:1–7.

CROCKER, T. T., and BENNETT, B. M. 1952. J. Immunol., **69**:183–93.

DAVIDSON, J. N. 1960. The biochemistry of the nucleic acids. 4th ed. London: Methuen & Co., Ltd.

DAVIS, D. J., and VOGEL, J. E. 1949. Proc. Soc. Exper. Biol. Med., **70**: 585–87.

DEMEREC, M. 1948. J. Bact., **56**:63–74.

EAGLE, H. 1955a. J. Biol. Chem., **214**:839-52.

———. 1955b. J. Exper. Med., **102**:595–600.

EARLY, R. L., and MORGAN, H. R. 1946. J. Immunol., **53**:251–57.

EATON, M. 1950. Ann. Rev. Microbiol., **4**:223–46.

FINDLAY, G. M. 1940. Brit. J. Exper. Path., **21**:356–60.

GAYLORD, W. H. 1954. J. Exper. Med., **100**:575-80.

GOGOLAK, F. M. 1953. J. Infect. Dis., **92**:248–53.

———. 1954. *Ibid.*, **95**:220–25.

GOGOLAK, F. M., and ROSS, M. R. 1955. Virology, **1**:474–96.

GOLUB, O. 1948. J. Lab. Clin. Med., **33**:1241–48.

GORDON, F. B., ANDREW, V. W., and WAGNER, J. C. 1957. Virology, **4**: 156–71.

GREENLAND, R. M. 1961. J. Infect. Dis., **108**:287–92.

HAHN, F. E., and CIAK, J. 1957. Science, **125**:119–20.

HAMRE, D., and RAKE, G. 1947. J. Infect. Dis., **81**:175–90.

HIGASHI, N. 1959. Ann. Rept. Inst. Virus Res. Kyoto Univ. (Ser. B), **2**: 1–21.

HILLEMAN, M. R., HAIG, D. A., and HELMHOLD, R. J. 1951. J. Immunol., **66**:115–30.

HOAGLAND, M. B. 1960. *In:* The nucleic acids, Vol. 3, ed. E. CHARGAFF and J. N. DAVIDSON, pp. 349–408. New York: Academic Press, Inc.

HUANG, C., and EATON, M. D. 1949. J. Bact., **58**:73–88.

HUENNEKINS, F. M., OSBORN, M. J., and WHITELEY, H. R. 1958. Science, **128**:120–24.

HURST, E. W. 1953. Brit. Med. Bull., **9**:180–85.

HURST, E. W., LANDQUIST, J. K., MELVIN, P., PETERS, J. M., SENIOR, N., SILK, J. A., and STACEY, G. J. 1953. Brit. J. Pharmacol. Chemotherap., **8**:297–305.

JENKIN, H. M. 1960. J. Bact., **80**:639–47.

JENKIN, H. M., ROSS, M. R., and MOULDER, J. W. 1961. J. Immunol., **86**: 123–27.

LAZARUS, A. S., and MEYER, K. F. 1939. J. Bact., **38**:121–51.

LEDERBERG, J. 1957. J. Bact., **73**:144.

LITWIN, J. 1959. J. Infect. Dis., **105**:129–60.

———. 1962. Ann. N.Y. Acad. Sc., in press.

LITWIN, J., OFFICER, J. E., BROWN, A., and MOULDER, J. W. 1961. J. Infect. Dis., **109**:251–79.

LOOSLI, C. G., HAMRE, D., GRAYSTON, J. T., and ALEXANDER, E. R. 1955. Antibiotics Ann., 1954–1955, pp. 490–503.

MACCALLUM, F. O. 1936. Brit. J. Exper. Path., **17**:472–81.

McQUILLEN, K. 1960. *In:* The bacteria, Vol. 1, ed. I. C. GUNSALUS and R. Y. STANIER, pp. 249–360. New York: Academic Press, Inc.

MANDELSTAM, J. 1960. Bact. Rev., 24:289–308.

MANIRE, G. P., and GALASSO, G. J. 1961. J. Immunol., 83:529–33.

MANIRE, G. P., and MEYER, K. F. 1950. J. Infect. Dis., 86:226–50.

MANIRE, G. P., and SMITH, K. O. 1959. J. Bact., 78:523–27.

MEYER, K. F. 1953. Ann. N.Y. Acad. Sc., 56:545–56.

———. 1958. *In:* Viral and rickettsial infections of man, ed. T. M. RIVERS and F. L. HORSFALL, JR., pp. 701–28. 3d ed. Philadelphia: J. B. Lippincott Co.

MEYER, K. F., and EDDIE, B. 1951. J. Infect. Dis., 88:109–25.

MITSUI, Y., SUZUKI, A., HANABUSA, J., MINODA, R., and OGOTA, S. 1957. Am. J. Ophth., 43:952–59.

MITSUI, Y., SUZUKI, A., HANABUSA, J., MINODA, R., OGOTA, S., FUKUSHIMA, S., and MINURA, M. 1958. Virology, 6:137–49.

MORGAN, H. R. 1948. J. Exper. Med., 88:285–94.

———. 1952. *Ibid.*, 95:269–76.

———. 1956. *Ibid.*, 103:37–47.

MORGAN, H. R., and BADER, J. C. 1957. J. Exper. Med., 106:39–44.

MOULDER, J. W. 1962. Ann. N.Y. Acad. Sc., in press.

MOULDER, J. W., COLÓN, J. I., RUDA, J., and ZEBOVITZ, M. M. 1956. J. Infect. Dis., 98:229–38.

MOULDER, J. W., McCORMACK, B. R. S., GOGOLAK, F. M., ZEBOVITZ, M. M., and ITATANI, M. K. 1955. J. Infect. Dis., 96:57–74.

MOULDER, J. W., McCORMACK, B. R. S., and ITATANI, M. K. 1953. J. Infect. Dis., 93:140–49.

MOULDER, J. W., RUDA, J., COLÓN, J. I., and GREENLAND, R. M. 1958. J. Infect. Dis., 102:186–201.

MOULDER, J. W., and WEISS, E. 1951a. J. Infect. Dis., 88:56–67.

———. 1951b. *Ibid.*, pp. 68–76.

OFFICER, J. E., and BROWN, A. 1960. J. Infect. Dis., 107:283–99.

———. 1961. Virology, 14:88–99.

PARK, J. T., and STROMINGER, J. L. 1957. Science, 125:99–101.

PELC, S. R., and CROCKER, T. T. 1961. Biochem. J., 79:20P.

PERRIN, J. 1952. J. Gen. Microbiol., 6:143–48.

POLLARD, M., STARR, T. J., TANAMI, Y., and ELLIOTT, A. Y. 1960. Proc. Soc. Exper. Biol. Med., 105:476–78.

RAKE, G., and JONES, H. P. 1942. J. Exper. Med., 75:323–37.

———. 1944. *Ibid.*, 79:463–86.

RICE, C. E. 1936. Am. J. Ophth., 19:1–8.

ROSS, M. R., and GOGOLAK, F. M. 1957. Virology, 3:365–73.

ROSS, M. R., and JENKIN, H. M. 1962. Ann. N.Y. Acad. Sc., in press.

SALTON, M. R. 1960. *In:* The bacteria, Vol. 1, ed. I. C. GUNSALUS and R. Y. STANIER, pp. 97–152. New York: Academic Press, Inc.

SMITH, K. O., and MANIRE, G. P. 1959. Proc. Soc. Exper. Biol. Med., **100:** 543–46.

STROMINGER, J. L., PARK, J. T., and THOMPSON, R. E. 1959. J. Biol. Chem., **234:**3263–68.

STUMPF, P. K. 1960. Ann. Rev. Biochem., **29:**261–94.

SWAIN, R. H. A. 1955. Brit. J. Exper. Path., **36:**507–14.

TAJIMA, M., NOMURA, Y., and KUBOTA, Y. 1957. J. Bact., **74:**605–20.

TAJIMA, M., SAMEJIMA, T., and NOMURA, Y. 1959. J. Bact., **77:**23–34.

TANAMI, Y., POLLARD, M., and STARR, T. J. 1961. Virology, **15:**22–29.

VOLKIN, E., and COHN, W. 1954. *In:* Methods of biochemical analysis, ed. D. GLICK, **1:**287–306. New York: Interscience Press, Inc.

WEISS, E. 1949. J. Infect. Dis., **84:**125–49.

———. 1950. *Ibid.,* **87:**249–63.

WEISS, E., and HUANG, J. S. 1954. J. Infect. Dis., **94:**107–25.

WOODROOFE, G. M., and MOULDER, J. W. 1960. J. Infect. Dis., **107:**195–202.

WOODS, D. D. 1940. Brit. J. Exper. Path., **21:**74–90.

———. 1952. Bull. World Health Org., **6:**35–57.

———. 1960. Proc. 4th Internat. Cong. Biochem., **11:**87–103.

WRIGHT, B. 1960. Proc. 4th Internat. Cong. Biochem., **11:**266–83.

YANAMURA, H. Y., and MEYER, K. F. 1941. J. Infect. Dis., **68:**1–15.

ZAHLER, S. A. 1953. J. Infect. Dis., **93:**150–58.

ZAHLER, S. A., and MOULDER, J. W. 1953. J. Infect. Dis., **93:**159–65.

CHAPTER V

The Pox Viruses

The best-known pox viruses are those of smallpox, vaccinia, cowpox, mousepox, fowlpox, and myxoma (Fenner and Burnet, 1957). Their close relationship is shown by a near-identical morphology and by the ability of any one active virus to reactivate heat-inactivated particles of any other virus of the pox group (Hanafusa et al., 1959; Fenner and Woodroofe, 1960). They also share a tendency to invade the cells of the skin, where they multiply, with the production of the characteristic lesions giving the pox group its name.

Three subgroups may be recognized on the basis of antigenic similarities. The members of each subgroup cross-react extensively with each other but not with members of the other two. The viruses of smallpox (variola), vaccinia, cowpox, and mousepox (ectromelia) show a very close antigenic relationship in all the conventional tests of viral serology. Almost all the biochemical research on the pox viruses has been carried out with vaccinia virus, the virus commercially propagated in calves and sheep for use in vaccination against smallpox. Most present-day vaccinia strains were probably derived from cowpox virus some time after the widespread adoption of Jennerian vaccination. Smallpox is an ancient disease of man and, in its classic, virulent form, an acute and highly lethal infection. In recent times, a mild form of smallpox, alastrim, has become prevalent, but the more acute form still persists. It is endemic in many regions of Asia and Africa, and occasional explosive outbreaks still occur in Western

Europe and North America. Fowlpox virus is the best-known representative of a large group of as yet ill-defined avian pox viruses which produce proliferative skin lesions in a variety of birds. Myxomatosis is a naturally occurring benign disease of New World rabbits which produces a highly lethal disease in Old World rabbits in the laboratory and when deliberately released in the field, as it has been in Europe and Australia. Myxoma virus is antigenically related to rabbit fibroma and squirrel fibroma viruses. There are a number of other viruses whose infectious particles closely resemble those of accepted members of the pox-virus group and which may eventually be included within the fold. The use of the heterologous reactivation phenomenon should be of decisive value in the taxonomy of the pox viruses.

Pox viruses are naturally transmitted from host to host by direct transfer of infective material, usually by the respiratory route, or by transmission by mosquitos or other arthropods. However, arthropod transmission of the pox viruses is entirely mechanical, and no growth or development of the infective agent occurs in the arthropod vector as it does in malaria or in rickettsial diseases.

GROWTH AND MORPHOLOGY

Growth of Pox Viruses in Experimental Systems

The first experimental system for cultivating pox viruses was the scarified skin of calves used for making vaccinia virus for smallpox vaccination. This method was adapted to the laboratory and used with great success in early studies on purified vaccinia virus. Quantitative methods for following the growth of pox viruses date from 1931, when Woodruff and Goodpasture grew fowlpox virus on the chorioallantoic membranes of chick embryos. It was soon demonstrated, particularly by Burnet (1936), that, under proper conditions, one infective particle produces one lesion, or pock, on the chorioallantoic membrane. Thus a pock count gives the number of infective particles in the inoculum.

Tissue-culture techniques are now widely used for studying the growth of pox viruses. These agents grow well in many of the commonly used cell lines, and most of them can be assayed by the plaque technique of Dulbecco (1952), in which one infective particle produces a discrete visible area of dead cells on a tissue-culture monolayer. The pox viruses characteristically show little tendency to be released from their host cells, and, for purposes of titration, it is necessary to disrupt the cells, usually by sonic or ultrasonic vibration.

In studies on morphology and growth, vaccinia virus has been used to the virtual exclusion of other members of the pox group. However, information is now accumulating on other viruses, and it appears that the results with vaccinia virus are generally representative of the entire group. Extensive references to studies with other pox viruses are given by Peters (1959).

Morphology of Isolated Particles

Crude preparations of infected tissues and highly purified vaccinia virus suspensions contain a particle utterly unlike any normal cell particle. That this distinctive body is the infectious particle of vaccinia has been demonstrated by many workers (see especially Smadel *et al.*, 1939; Kaplan and Valentine, 1959; Overman and Sharp, 1959). In air-dried preparations examined with the electron microscope, the elementary bodies of vaccinia are about 230 mμ in length and look like little bricks with rounded corners (Fig. V-1). There is an electron-dense central body and smaller masses of lesser density at the four corners (Green *et al.*, 1942). The central body has the shape of a dumbbell oriented along the long axis of the particle (Peters, 1956).

Dawson and McFarlane (1948) found that vaccinia ele-

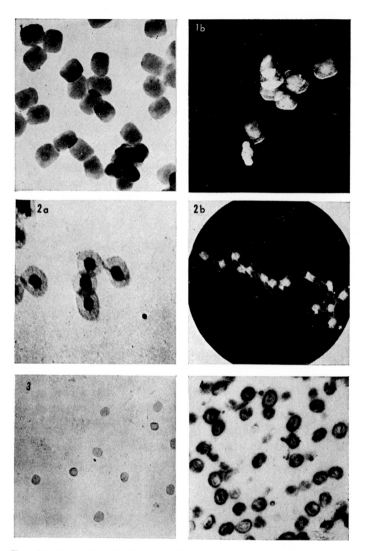

FIGS. V-1–V-4.—Fig. V-1: Vaccinia virus purified by salt flocculation and fixed with osmic acid. 1a, unshadowed; 1b, shadowed with gold. Both 27,500×. From Dawson and McFarlane (1948). Reproduced by permission the authors and *Nature*. Fig. V-2: Same as Fig. 1, but after peptic digestion. Fig. V-3: Empty membranes of vaccinia virus produced by treatment of osmic acid–fixed elementary bodies with 0.02 per cent papain at pH 7 in the presence of 0.1 M cysteine. This produces the same effect as that of treatment with pepsin, DNase, and pepsin again. 10,000×. This is a previously unpublished electron micrograph reproduced here through the kindness of Professor D. Peters. Fig. V-4: Section through a pellet of vaccinia virus purified by the fluorocarbon method. Fixed with potassium permanganate and imbedded in methacrylate. 18,500×. From Epstein (1958). Reproduced by permission of the author and the *British Journal of Experimental Pathology*.

mentary bodies were attacked by pepsin at pH 3, with dissolution of most of the viral substance. There was left behind an electron-dense central body surrounded by a less dense membrane (Fig. V-2). All the viral DNA remained in the pepsin-resistant structure and could be brought into solution with deoxyribonuclease (DNase), but there was no accompanying change in the appearance of the residual structure. However, Peters and Stoeckenius (1954) showed that the nuclease treatment had rendered the central body pepsin-sensitive. Thus, if elementary bodies were exposed in succession to pepsin, DNase, and pepsin again, only collapsed and empty membranes remained (Fig. V-3). The picture obtained by enzymic dissection has been confirmed by examination of thin sections of fixed pellets of purified elementary bodies (Peters, 1956; Epstein, 1958) (Fig. V-4). These results suggest that the elementary body consists of a pepsin-resistant enveloping membrane surrounding a pepsin-sensitive protein area, in the center of which is a core of deoxyribonucleoprotein which is attacked by pepsin only after the nucleic acid is depolymerized by its specific nuclease. The membrane has been analogized to the bacterial cell wall, but there is little information as to its chemical composition. It does not contain muramic acid (Allison and Perkins, 1960).

Intracellular Development

Although the growth of viruses of the pox group had been thoroughly studied with the light microscope by such workers as Bland and Robinow (1939), most of our present concepts of the growth of vaccinia and related agents have arisen from study of thin sections of infected tissues with the electron microscope. The observations of Morgan and Wykoff (1950), Bang (1950), Wykoff (1951), Gaylord and Melnick (1953), Morgan *et al.* (1954, 1955), Flewett (1956), Andres *et al.* (1958), Peters (1960), and Higashi and his associates (see Higashi, 1959, for references) are in broad general agreement, and from them emerges the following picture of the multiplication of vaccinia virus.

The host systems most frequently used have been the chorioallantoic ectoderm of the chick embryo or monolayers of HeLa cells. For about 6–8 hours after infection, no structures recognizable as virus particles or as being related to virus particles can be seen. During this period, intracellular infectivity remains low and constant, and there are probably no intact intracellular infectious particles present at all.

The first recognizable morphologic change occurs about 6 hours after infection, when a region of high electron density appears in the cytoplasm. It is usually located near the nucleus and is referred to as "matrix" or "viroplasm." Shortly thereafter the first virus particles appear in the matrix. These are the developmental or immature bodies (Fig. V-5). They appear as ellipsoids with axes of about 0.2 and 0.3 μ, but they are probably actually round bodies distorted along one axis by the knife of the ultramicrotome. The developmental body characteristically has a single limiting membrane inclosing a granular viroplasm and a dense, oval, central body. The words "immature" and "developmental" are misnomers. These bodies are clearly infective because the intracellular infectivity titer begins to rise when these bodies are the only virus structures present.

The so-called mature bodies do not appear until about 15 hours after infection. They arise through internal rearrangement of developmental bodies, and numerous transitional forms may be seen. Mature bodies are seen first intracytoplasmically and later extracellularly (Fig. V-6). The extracellular titer always lags behind the intracellular titer, indicating that the virus of vaccinia is released from the cell slowly and incompletely. The final "mature" elementary body is somewhat larger than the "immature" body, with axes of about 0.2 and 0.35 μ. It has a distinct double membrane and an inner body of variable shape. The mature body is the

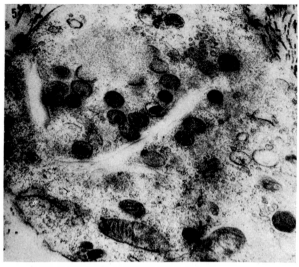

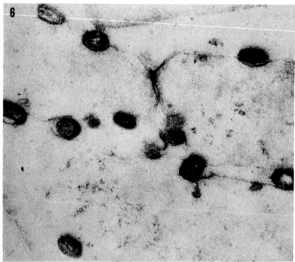

Figs. V-5–V-6.—Fig. V-5: Fowlpox virus in the chorioallantoic membrane. Thin section prepared by fixing in osmic acid and imbedding in methacrylate. Developmental bodies in what is apparently a cytoplasmic center of viral synthesis (*upper left*). 20,000×. From Morgan *et al.* (1954). Reproduced by permission of the authors and the *Journal of Experimental Medicine*. Fig. V-6: Like Fig. 5. A late stage in fowlpox virus reproduction, showing mature elementary bodies in the extracellular spaces. 30,000×.

major type present in purified preparations subjected to enzymic dissection and chemical analysis.

The multiplication of vaccinia virus differs in two major
respects from the reproductive mechanisms previously described for plasmodia, rickettsiae, and members of the psittacosis group. First, immediately after infection there occurs
a period during which no intact virus particles may be seen
within the host cell. Second, once recognizable virus particles
appear, they are never seen to multiply by binary fission or
by any other mechanism. Developmental bodies become mature bodies, but neither type of body gives rise to more virus
particles. These two phenomena are obviously related and
point to a reproductive mechanism for the pox group entirely
unlike those of the other intracellular parasites we have been
considering. This is, of course, the viral mode of multiplication defined in chapter i, and in a later section of this chapter
we shall consider in detail the evidence for its occurrence in
vaccinia virus.

Inhibition of Multiplication by Chemotherapeutic Agents

The multiplication of vaccinia virus and other members of
the pox group is not inhibited by any of the common antibiotics and other chemotherapeutic agents active against
bacteria, the rickettsiae, and the psittacosis group. This
again indicates a fundamental difference between the multiplication of the pox viruses and the other obligate intracellular parasites. Vaccinia virus multiplication is inhibited by a
number of chemicals (see Horsfall, 1959; Staehelin, 1959),
but their mode of action is unknown.

CHEMICAL COMPOSITION OF ISOLATED VIRUS PARTICLES

Vaccinia virus was the first animal virus obtained in highly
purified form and subjected to exhaustive physical and chemical analysis (reviewed in detail by Smadel and Hoagland,

1942). This work was of critical importance in characterizing the pox-virus group and was probably of even greater importance in its general influence on subsequent work with other animal viruses, the psittacosis group, and the rickettsiae. None of the other pox viruses has been studied in comparable detail, but they are all probably similar to vaccinia virus in chemical composition.

Preparation of Purified Suspensions

The classic preparation of vaccinia virus begins with dermal pulp harvested from confluent cutaneous lesions in rabbits (Ledingham, 1931; Craigie, 1932; Craigie and Wishart, 1934; McFarlane *et al.*, 1939; Hoagland *et al.*, 1940). The essence of the method is the infection of large numbers of cells in the skin of rabbits and the harvesting of the virus-laden contents of the infected cells without also obtaining large amounts of cellular debris. The dermal pulp so obtained is subjected to several cycles of differential centrifugation to yield the final purified suspension.

A second method consists of homogenizing confluently infected chorioallantoic membranes or heavily infected cell cultures with a fluorocarbon (Gessler *et al.*, 1956; Epstein, 1958).[1] After fluorocarbon homogenization, the elementary bodies are found in the aqueous phase, while most of the host-cell material is left behind in the fluorocarbon phase or at the interface. Satisfactory preparations are obtained by two to four repetitions of this procedure. Flocculation with M sodium chloride followed by redispersion with sonic or ultrasonic vibrations was introduced by Dawson and McFarlane (1948) as a useful final step in purification.

Criteria of Purity

Vaccinial preparations obtained by differential centrifugation of infected dermal pulp have been rigorously examined

---

[1] Such as 1-dichlorofluoro-2-difluorochloroethane.

by a variety of techniques. Chemical analysis of different lots of virus gave highly reproducible results, while physical measurements revealed a single boundary in the analytical ultracentrifuge (Pickels and Smadel, 1938; Smadel *et al.*, 1938) and in the Tiselius electrophoresis apparatus (McFarlane, 1940; Shedlovsky and Smadel, 1940). Smadel *et al.* (1939) calculated the weight of a single elementary body from size and density data obtained with the ultracentrifuge and thus determined the number of elementary bodies in several dried purified preparations whose pock counts had been determined before drying. The ratio of total elementary bodies to pock counts approached unity. All these results indicated that the vaccinia preparations were of a high order of purity, a conclusion directly confirmed when similar preparations were examined with the electron microscope and found to consist almost exclusively of elementary bodies of characteristic morphology (Green *et al.*, 1942).

The virus obtained by fluorocarbon treatment is free of complement-fixing host antigens (Hamparian *et al.*, 1958) and formed host elements (Epstein, 1958). However, it contains an amorphous phase consisting mainly of DNA and polysaccharide (Holt and Epstein, 1958). The latter authors recommend treating fluorocarbon-prepared virus with deoxyribonuclease.

Basic Constituents

Vaccinia virus is almost as complex in chemical composition as are rickettsiae or members of the psittacosis group and has been analyzed more thoroughly than either of these groups of agents.

The most important chemical difference between the pox viruses and the other intracellular parasites discussed in previous chapters is that they almost certainly contain only one kind of nucleic acid, DNA. The presence of DNA in vaccinia virus was first reported by McFarlane and Macfarlane

(1939) and McFarlane *et al.* (1939). Hoagland, Lavin, Smadel, and Rivers (1940) carefully studied the nucleic acid of vaccinia virus with the best methods then available and concluded that this agent contained 5.6 per cent DNA and little or no RNA. Their conclusions have been confirmed by the use of more sensitive modern methods (Wyatt and Cohen, 1953; Pfau and McCrea, 1961; Randall *et al.*, 1961). If RNA is present, it must be in very low concentration.

The base ratios reported by Wyatt and Cohn and Randall *et al.* are consonant with the double-stranded DNA structure of Watson and Crick (molar ratios of adenine to thymine and guanine to cytosine of near unity). However, Pfau and McCrea found that the behavior of vaccinial DNA toward formaldehyde and heat to be highly suggestive of a single-stranded molecule. Clarification of the detailed structure of the pox group DNA is needed.

Vaccinia virus contains about 6 per cent lipid, made up of approximately equal parts of neutral fat, phospholipid, and cholesterol (Hoagland, Smadel, and Rivers, 1940). The cholesterol could be extracted with ether without loss of infectivity, but the neutral fat and phospholipid were extracted only with alcohol-ether mixtures, and complete inactivation resulted (McFarlane *et al.*, 1939; Hoagland, Smadel, and Rivers, 1940). Pancreatic lipase did not attack the neutral fat in intact elementary bodies, although it readily hydrolyzed the extracted lipid. It thus appears that neutral fat and phospholipid are necessary for infectivity, while cholesterol is not. However, this does not necessarily mean that the cholesterol is just a host-derived contaminant.

If the total nitrogen unaccounted for by other nitrogen-containing constituents is all protein nitrogen, then vaccinia elementary bodies are almost 90 per cent protein (McFarlane *et al.*, 1939; Hoagland, Smadel, and Rivers, 1940). However, the α-amino nitrogen value suggests a protein content only one-third as large (Hoagland, Smadel, and Rivers, 1940). Amino acid analyses are not available.

Vaccinia virus contains about 3 per cent total acid-hydrolyzable reducing sugar, most of which can be accounted for by the deoxyribose of the DNA (McFarlane *et al.*, 1939; Hoagland, Smadel, and Rivers, 1940). A small amount of hexoseamine is also present (McFarlane *et al.*, 1939; Smadel *et al.*, 1940).

Enzymes and Coenzymes

Cytochrome oxidase and cytochromes (Hoagland *et al.*, 1941*a*), a variety of dehydrogenases (Macfarlane and Salaman, 1938; Macfarlane and Dolby, 1940; Hoagland *et al.*, 1942), and several enzymes of the glycolytic cycle (Macfarlane and Dolby, 1940) were all tested for in heavy suspensions of vaccinial elementary bodies, and all were absent. Thus it appears unlikely that vaccinia virus has independent energy-yielding enzyme systems.

However, the search for respiratory enzymes did reveal the presence of significant concentrations of copper (Hoagland *et al.*, 1941*a*) and flavinadenine dinucleotide (Hoagland *et al.*, 1941*b*) in purified preparations. Both substances were firmly bound to the elementary bodies and were not dissociated by procedures which should have disrupted the loose binding of the free compounds. Likewise, both copper and flavin were concentrated several fold during the course of virus purification. Attempts to show that they acted as the coenzymes of electron-transporting enzymes were not successful.

Biotin was also found in vaccinia virus by Hoagland, Ward, Smadel, and Rivers (1940). Some was free, but there was a fourfold increase in the biotin available for growth of *Clostridium butylicum* after acid or alkali hydrolysis. Lynen *et al.* (1959) have shown that biotin is the coenzyme for the enzymic addition of carbon dioxide to β-methyl-glutacanyl-

Co A and have suggested a general role for biotin in reactions of carboxylation (see also Ochoa and Kaziro, 1961). How biotin could perform a similar function in vaccinia virus is not clear.

Preparations of purified vaccinia virus exhibited phosphatase, catalase, and lipase activity (Macfarlane and Salaman, 1938; Macfarlane and Dolby, 1940; Hoagland *et al.*, 1942). However, elementary bodies adsorb these highly active enzymes (but not a number of others) from dilute solution, and they are probably of host-cell origin (Hoagland *et al.*, 1942).

In summary, although purified preparations of vaccinia virus contain a number of enzymes and coenzymes, all of them are also found in the host cell in which the virus grows, and none can be assigned a definite role in virus multiplication. This does not mean that they are not integral virus components, but it does mean that it will be exceedingly difficult to prove that they are.

Multiplication of Pox Viruses

We have just seen that the pox viruses exhibit no enzymic activities with any obvious relation to their multiplication and that existing virus particles show no indication of giving rise to additional particles. It has therefore been necessary to study pox-virus multiplication in terms of the events taking taking place in infected cells.

Eclipse of the Infecting Particles

When mature infectious particles are incubated with susceptible cell cultures for 1 hour at 37° C., electron microscopy of thin sections reveals many particles of mature structure adsorbed to the host-cell surfaces and occasional particles deep in the cytoplasm (Higashi *et al.*, 1960). Thereafter, it is generally agreed by all investigators that no recognizable intracellular virus particles may be found until new particles, with the structure of developmental virus, appear approximately 5 hours later. What occurs in the infected cell during this morphologically blank period is of critical importance in understanding how the pox viruses reproduce themselves.

Because there has existed for a number of years a large and detailed body of knowledge concerning the mode of reproduction of bacterial viruses (see Adams, 1959), the multiplication of other viruses is inevitably compared, sometimes consciously and sometimes unconsciously, with that of the bacterial viruses. Although it is really much more complicated, the bacteriophage particle is, at first approximation, a core of DNA surrounded by a coat of protein. The protein coat adsorbs to the bacterial surface, and a special mechanism injects the DNA into the bacterium, destroying in the process the integrity of the infecting particle. The injected DNA brings about a complete reorganization of the enzymic machinery of the host. A number of new enzymes are synthesized, and the reorganized cell synthesizes phage DNA and protein, which are ultimately assembled into new infective phage particles. The period from the injection of the DNA until the appearance of the first complete new particle is marked by the entire absence of intracellular infectivity and has been called the "eclipse period."

The small animal viruses consisting of an RNA core and a protein coat, such as polio virus and the encephalitis viruses, reproduce by a roughly analogous mechanism (see Isaacs, 1959). The entire infective particle penetrates the host cytoplasm, where the protein coat is shed and the viral RNA assumes control of host biosynthetic potentialities. The demonstration that the RNA of animal and plant viruses (Schuster, 1960) and the DNA of bacteriophages (Guthrie and Sinsheimer, 1960; Meyer *et al.*, 1961) are of themselves infectious and capable of producing complete progeny gives final proof of the multiplication of these viruses in the form of their naked nucleic acids. This mode of reproduction has been taken as the principal criterion for the viral nature of an infectious agent as opposed to an organismal one (Lwoff, 1957, 1959).

Early attempts to demonstrate an eclipse phase in the multiplication of vaccinia virus were complicated by the difficulty of distinguishing between true intracellular virus and unadsorbed or unpenetrated virus from the inoculum (reviewed by Isaacs, 1959). Furness and Youngner (1959) and Postlethwaite and Maitland (1960) circumvented this difficulty by using cell-culture techniques. Figure V-7 gives an idealized version of the growth curve of vaccinia virus in cell culture. It may be referred to in the discussion to follow as

UNITS OF INFECTIVE VIRUS

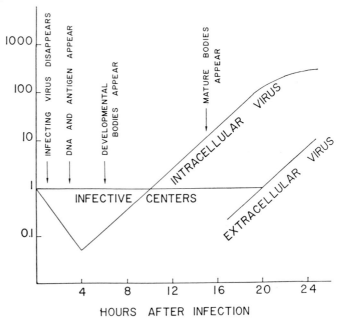

Fig. V-7.—An idealized growth curve for vaccinia virus. The vertical scale is based on an assumption of the adsorption of one infectious unit of virus by one host cell.

142

a means of keeping the sequence of various important events clearly in mind. Cell cultures were allowed to adsorb vaccinia virus, excess inoculum was washed out, and at frequent intervals two kinds of infectivity determinations were made. In the first, the host cells were disintegrated and plated on cell sheets to give plaque counts equivalent to the number of intracellular infective particles present. In the second, whole intact cells were plated. These gave plaque counts equal to the number of infective centers, that is, the number of cells eventually capable of producing mature infectious virus and thus initiating plaque formation. The number of infective centers remained constant throughout the first cycle of growth, but the intracellular virus titer fell to a minimum at about 4 hours and then rose logarithmically until about 300 infective particles per cell had been formed at 20 hours. However, at 4 hours after infection, there were fifteen to thirty times as many infective centers as intracellular virus particles. Thus infectious particles could be detected in only one out of every 15–30 cells which eventually produced a new generation of virus. This is one way of saying that an eclipse phase occurs in the multiplication of vaccinia virus and, we assume, the other pox viruses as well.

Easterbrook (1961) has confirmed the existence of an eclipse phase by studying single KB cells infected with vaccinia virus. Between 1 and 5 hours after infection, 9 out of 10 cells acted as infective centers, while only 1 out of 25 contained infectious intracellular virus.

Initiation of Multiplication

If, in the hours immediately following infection of a cell with vaccinia virus, intracellular infectious units cannot be found in a high proportion of the cells which eventually produce virus, then these cells must, at that time, contain viral units smaller than the infectious unit itself. The analogy with

bacteriophage suggests that these subunits are vaccinial DNA and vaccinial protein and that it should be possible to detect the subunits before new infectious particles begin to appear in the host cell. Noyes and Watson (1955) first used fluorescent antibody for visualization of virus antigen, presumably protein. Several workers have demonstrated the synthesis of vaccinial DNA by feeding tritiated thymidine to infected cells and locating the thymidine incorporated into DNA by autoradiographs (Magee *et al.*, 1960; Cairns, 1960; Sheek and Magee, 1961; Yamamoto and Black, 1961). Since cell cultures synthesize nuclear DNA only during the third quarter of interphase (Firket and Verly, 1958) and do not make DNA in the cytoplasm at all, the uptake of H^3-thymidine into the cytoplasmic virus inclusions may be clearly observed. We shall assume in the discussion to follow that vaccinia virus consists of a protein coat and a DNA center, although we have already seen that such an assumption involves even more simplification for vaccinia virus than for bacteriophage. For the moment, let us beg the question as to whether such drastic simplification is justified.

The studies of Cairns (1960) are especially informative because he employed a technique that allowed visualization of both protein (fluorescent antibody) and DNA (H^3-thymidine) in one and the same cell. After vaccinia virus had been adsorbed on a monolayer of KB cells, viral DNA and protein appeared at the same time and in the same discrete loci near the nuclear membrane. The lag between detection of the viral subunits and infection of the cells was about 3.5 hours.

Other workers have also observed that DNA synthesis starts at about this time. Sheek and Magee (1961) and Yamamoto and Black (1961) employed techniques similar to those of Cairns and also saw viral DNA for the first time at about 3.5 hours after infection. Magee *et al.* (1960) quantitatively measured the uptake of H^3-thymidine into vaccinial DNA

and found maximum incorporation 3.5–6 hours after infection. Salzman (1960) used 5-fluorodeoxyuridine, which inhibits DNA synthesis by preventing the conversion of deoxyuridilic acid to thymidilic acid but does not prevent the formation of infective virus from DNA that had been synthesized before the inhibitor was added. By comparing the amount of infectious virus formed in cell cultures to which 5-fluorodeoxyuridine had been added at different times after infection, he concluded that the formation of infective virus lagged 4–6 hours behind the synthesis of DNA, most of which was formed 2.5–6 hours after the virus entered the cell.

Loh and Riggs (1961) used immunofluorescent techniques to confirm that viral antigen appeared in the cytoplasm of HeLa cells infected with vaccinia virus at about the same time as did viral DNA. By employing specific antisera, they showed further that, of the various distinct vaccinial antigens, the LS antigen appeared at 4 hours, while the nucleoprotein antigen could be detected only after 5–6 hours. Although both antigens appeared in the perinuclear region, Loh and Riggs could distinguish their centers of synthesis, and intimate mixing did not occur until about 8 hours after infection, when the intracellular infectivity had begun to rise. The significance of these antigens in the architecture of the virus particle is not clearly understood. The LS antigen is a simple protein, while the nucleoprotein antigen contains 6 per cent DNA (Smadel and Hoagland, 1942). Both are probably surface antigens because their antibodies agglutinate intact virus particles.

Cairns (1960) made two other important observations concerning the initiation of infection. First, in cells infected with several virus particles, each one sets up a separate center of virus synthesis, and all centers begin to produce virus at the same time. Second, the more infecting particles per cell, the sooner that cell will start producing virus until the minimum

delay of 3.5 hours between infection and the appearance of DNA and antigen is reached. He believes that, among the several infecting particles, only one, the initiator, starts the chain of events leading to virus reproduction. The act of initiation begins a preparatory period of 3–4 hours, at the end of which all centers begin to produce virus at the same time. If each invading particle has a constant probability of initiating infection, then the more particles per cell, the greater the chance of initiation in any given interval.

The nature of the act of initiation is unknown. It could involve the production of a substance vital to virus synthesis or the destruction of an inhibitor which prevents it. Whatever the nature of initiation, it is of fundamental importance that all centers of synthesis begin operating at the same time. This strongly suggests that a generalized reorganization of the host cytoplasm has occurred. It is in sharp contrast to the appearance of cells multiply infected with members of the psittacosis group in which both early and late vesicles may be seen side by side (see, for example, Officer and Brown, 1960, 1961).

Source of the Viral DNA

All workers agree that the nuclear DNA of the host cell is not used for synthesis of viral DNA. Magee *et al.* (1959) infected HeLa cells previously labeled with H^3-thymidine and found none of the label in the new virus. Both Cairns (1960) and Yamamoto and Black (1961) observed nuclear DNA being formed long after infection, while Noyes and Watson (1955) observed infected cells in mitosis.

There is also agreement that viral DNA is synthesized in the cytoplasm and not in the nucleus (Cairns, 1960; Sheek and Magee, 1961; Yamamoto and Black, 1961). A puzzling observation was made by Sheek and Magee. During the first 2 hours after infection, they saw intranuclear inclusion bodies

which later migrated to the cytoplasm and became centers of DNA synthesis.

The rapid incorporation of thymidine into vaccinial DNA shows that it is synthesized from low-molecular-weight components. The 3–4-hour interval between infection and first appearance of viral DNA probably represents the time necessary for production of the new metabolic machinery required for making a foreign species of DNA in the cytoplasm. Infected cells show an increased rate of incorporation of adenine (Joklik, 1959; Joklik and Rodrick, 1959) and of inorganic phosphate (Nishimura and Tagaya, 1959) into ribosomal RNA. Tamm and Bablanian (1960) have reported that RNase inhibits multiplication of vaccinia virus. One is tempted to interpret these observations in terms of the synthesis of new RNA essential for the production of viral DNA and protein.

There has been considerable speculation about how the pox viruses induce their host cells to make DNA in the cytoplasm, a synthesis restricted to the nucleus in uninfected cells. The recently formulated "messenger RNA" theory of Jacob and Monod (1961), which is supported by experiments on uninfected (Gros *et al.*, 1961) and phage-infected (Brenner *et al.*, 1961) *Escherichia coli*, offers a hint as to how this can occur. According to the messenger theory, the information for the synthesis of proteins is carried from the nucleus to the ribosomes by a special kind of short-lived, unstable RNA, called "messenger RNA." Thus the theory ascribes an entirely non-specific role to the RNA of the ribosomes and assumes all specific RNA to be of nuclear origin. In infection with a virulent phage, one of the first acts of the phage DNA is to destroy the host DNA. Then, according to the messenger theory, phage DNA causes the synthesis of new messenger RNA with phage specificity. This RNA then replaces the host message to the ribosomes with one calling for synthesis of phage-specific protein.

These ideas suggest the possible events in vaccinia virus replication shown in Diagram V-1. The DNA of the infecting particle causes the synthesis of messenger RNA of viral specificity which is capable of instructing the host ribosomes to make viral protein by the same enzymatic mechanism that

DIAGRAM V-1

FORMULATION OF CYTOPLASMIC SYNTHESIS OF VIRAL PROTEIN AND DNA
ON BASIS OF MESSENGER THEORY OF JACOB AND MONOD

Uninfected Cell

$$\text{1) Amino Acids} \quad \xrightarrow[\text{Ribosomes}]{\overset{\text{RNA*}}{\text{host}}} \quad \underset{\text{host}}{\text{Protein}}$$

Infected Cell

$$\text{1) Ribonucleotides} \quad \xrightarrow[\text{(Nucleus?)}]{\overset{\text{DNA}}{\text{virus}}} \quad \underset{\text{virus}}{\text{RNA}}$$

$$\text{2)} \underset{\text{virus}}{\text{RNA}} \quad +\underset{\text{host}}{\text{RNA}}\text{——Ribosomes}\longrightarrow$$

$$\underset{\text{virus}}{\text{RNA}}\text{——Ribosomes}+\underset{\text{host}}{\text{RNA}}$$

$$\text{3}a\text{) Amino acids} \quad \xrightarrow[\text{Ribosomes}]{\overset{\text{RNA}}{\text{virus}}} \quad \underset{\text{virus}}{\text{Protein}}$$

$$\text{3}b\text{) Amino acids} \quad \xrightarrow[\text{Ribosomes}]{\overset{\text{RNA}}{\text{virus}}} \quad \underset{\text{DNA enzymes}}{\text{Protein}}$$

$$\text{4) Deoxyribonucleotides} \quad \xrightarrow[\underset{\text{virus}}{\text{(DNA} \quad \text{primer)}}]{\overset{\text{Protein}}{\text{DNA enzymes}}} \quad \underset{\text{virus}}{\text{DNA}}$$

* RNA always refers to messenger RNA.

they had previously used to make host protein. However, since synthesis of DNA does not occur in the cytoplasm, the enzyme proteins required for DNA formation are not known to be present. We must therefore assume that the viral messenger RNA instructs the ribosomes to make not only the proteins which appear in the infective particle but also the enzyme proteins required for synthesis of viral DNA. We must also assume that the viral messenger RNA can displace host messenger RNA from the ribosomes because the nucleus functions normally for a long time after infection. Once the substitution has occurred, the viral synthetic center is ready to operate. In the light of this hypothesis, the conclusion of Sheek and Magee (1961) that the invading particle proceeds directly to the nucleus and then re-enters the cytoplasm to initiate synthesis of new virus is particularly attractive, for it provides an opportunity for the viral messenger RNA to be synthesized in the nucleus at the same site as the host messenger RNA.

Appearance of Infective Virus

Cairns's technique shows that viral antigens and DNA appear in the same place in the cytoplasm at about the same time, but it does not show when they cease being separate entities and are assembled into morphologic units, and it does not tell whether infectivity first appears before or after the assembly. Treatment either of extracted intracellular infectivity or of intact infected cells with DNase has been used to estimate the time of incorporation of DNA into a virus particle. However, it is possible that immature developmental forms of virus may not possess the pepsin-sensitive, DNase-resistant outer layer possessed by mature particles (Dawson and McFarlane, 1948; Peters and Stoeckenius, 1954; Peters, 1956). Therefore, destruction of intracellular infectivity by DNase does not necessarily indicate the presence of infectious DNA. Similarly, labeled DNA in radioautographs which is lost upon exposure to DNase may already have been incorporated into a developmental particle. To add to the confusion, there is disagreement as to how much of the early infectivity and radioautographically visualized DNA is destroyed by the nuclease (compare Furness and Youngner, 1959; Cairns, 1960; Yamamoto and Black, 1961). Sheek (1961) has found that the nature of the infecting virus may profoundly affect the DNase sensitivity of its progeny. This may explain the divergent results. It should be pointed out here that infectious DNA has not yet been obtained from any pox virus.

Neutralization of infectivity with antibody offers another approach to the problem. Naked DNA should not be neutralized by antiserum, and a particle with an incomplete antigenic complement might be only partially neutralized. There appears to be a more or less constant fraction of intracellular infectivity neutralized by antiserum throughout the growth cycle of vaccinia virus (Sheek, 1961), suggesting early union of antigen and DNA.

Information about the assembly of the infective particle is therefore fragmentary and somewhat contradictory. However, when it is remembered that developmental particles may be seen only about 2 hours after DNA and antigen appear and that infectivity begins to rise soon thereafter, it seems reasonably certain that the viral subunits are assembled soon after synthesis into particles that are infective but may still lack a complete complement of enveloping membranes.

Maturation

As we have already seen, the change from developmental particle to mature particle involves morphologic alterations in both central structures and enveloping membranes. We may reason that these changes make the mature particle more resistant to the hostile agents it will encounter in reaching a new cell, but we know nothing about the underlying causes. Is maturation a spontaneous non-enzymatic rearrangement of existing structures, or is it the biosynthesis of new structures? If it is enzymatic, are the enzymes involved host enzymes or viral enzymes?

The maturation process has no counterpart in phages or in the RNA viruses, both of which are assembled in final form. It is somewhat reiminiscent of the changes in particle morphology late in the growth cycle of the psittacosis group.

Genetic Recombination

When the same cell is infected with a large number of two different pox viruses recognizably different in several characters, there are produced hybrid progeny with genomes indicative of extensive and orderly genetic recombination of their DNA (Fenner and Comben, 1958; Fenner, 1959; Gemmel and Cairns, 1959; Gemmel and Fenner, 1959; Woodroofe and Fenner, 1960). It is difficult to interpret pox-virus recombination in terms of the reproductive events just described. In analogy to recombination between bacterial viruses, recombination would be expected to occur in the eclipse period by matings between free DNA molecules. However, the radioautographic and fluorescent antibody studies clearly show that different sites of virus synthesis started by different infecting particles remain distinct for a long time and do not fuse until late in the growth cycle, when new viral DNA is being formed very slowly, if at all.

Reactivation of Heat-inactivated Pox Viruses

When Berry and Dedrick (1936) injected rabbits with a mixture of heat-inactivated myxoma virus and active fibroma virus, they recovered active myxoma virus. Since fibroma virus produces a benign infection in rabbits, while myxoma virus causes a uniformly fatal one, small amounts of active myxoma virus were readily detected. Berry and Dedrick considered this phenomenon to be analogous to the transformation of pneumococcal capsular types, which we now know to result from the transfer of a relatively small fragment of DNA from one pneumococcus to another. However, they also considered the possibility that the heat-killed myxoma virus might be reactivated by the unheated fibroma particles.

The results of Berry and Dedrick were soon confirmed, but study of the underlying mechanisms in intact animals was made impossible by the highly erratic nature of the results. Kilham's (1957) demonstration that the Berry-Dedrick phenomenon can be consistently obtained in cell cultures infected with heat-killed myxoma virus and active fibroma virus opened the way to analysis of the phenomenon. Even with the introduction of the cell culture as the medium in which the "transformation" occurred, still the only marker used was rabbit virulence. Fenner and his associates (Fenner *et al.*, 1959; Joklik, Woodroofe, Holmes, and Fenner, 1960) used virus strains with several independent genetic markers which they had obtained for their recombination studies. The extra markers allowed them to show that when a living virulent virus was recovered from an animal inoculated with a mixture of heat-inactivated virulent virus and active avirulent virus, some of the virulent clones resembled the original virulent virus in every respect, while other equally virulent clones had markers derived from both original viruses. The reappearance of virulent strains identical in every marker tested with the original heat-killed one is best interpreted as a reactivation of the heated virus by the unheated one. Recombination between their progeny would produce virulent progeny with some of the avirulent markers.

The nature of this reactivation has been clarified by studying the essential properties of the reactivating and the reactivated particle. The most efficient agents for producing reactivatible particles are heat and urea, both mild protein-denaturing agents (Shack and Kilham, 1959; Joklik, Holmes, and Briggs, 1960). It thus appears that such particles lack some native protein essential to initiation of multiplication, which must be supplied by the reactivating particle. Shack and Kilham (1959) have shown that if heat-inactivated myxoma virus is treated with urea, it may still be reactivated, but its biological activity is now destroyed by DNase. This indicates that if a particle is to be reactivated, it must have its DNA intact. Working from the other direction, Joklik, Abel, and Holmes (1960) treated the reactivating particle with nitrogen mustard, which destroys DNA but not protein, and found that its ability to reactivate heat-inactivated virus was unimpaired, thus showing that only protein, and not DNA, is required to cause reactivation.

However, it must not be concluded that the biological activity of the reactivatible particle is dependent solely on the preservation of its DNA. Heat-treated reactivatible particles are not DNase-sensitive, showing that the DNase-resistant protein layer already described is still present. Strong denaturing agents, such as sodium dodecylsulfate, and powerful proteinases, such as papain, destroy the ability to be reactivated by denaturing or digesting a protein essential for multiplication that cannot be supplied by the reactivating particle.

Thus the reactivation of heat-inactivated pox viruses is a non-genetic reaction involving a viral protein and not viral DNA. Since any active pox virus may reactivate any other heat-killed pox virus (Hanafusa *et al.*, 1959; Fenner and Woodroofe, 1960), this protein must be common to the entire pox group. Since the reactivation phenomenon cuts across the serologically distinct subgroups within the pox family, it must not be identical with any of the known pox-virus antigens. Cairns (1960) has pointed out the resemblance between the effect of active virus on heat-treated virus and the effect of the initiator on the other infecting particles in a multiply infected cell. It is highly probable that continued study of reactivation will be a fruitful approach to the understanding of the initial phases of pox-virus multiplication.

Pathogenesis of Pox-Virus Infections

All pox viruses produce essentially the same types of lesions, and all except molluscum contagiosum may give rise to generalized infections. Taking the studies of Fenner (1948, 1949) on the pathogenesis of ectromelia in the mouse as a model for the group, several stages of infection may be recognized. The invading virus sets up a primary site of multiplication in the skin (or respiratory tract); it spreads via the lymphatics and blood stream to the viscera, where extensive viral multiplication occurs; the new virus reinvades the blood stream and is carried to the skin, where it produces lesions typical of the disease. It is unfortunate that the wealth of chemical and morphologic information about the pox group cannot yet be effectively applied to the understanding of the diseases they produce and that the following discussion must therefore be a fragmentary one.

Invasion

We have already seen that, whatever the mechanism, the invasion of a cell by a pox virus may be a highly efficient process, with the ratio of total particles to infective units approaching 1. The results of Parker *et al.* (1941) show that the mechanism is also specific. They found that passage of vaccinia virus in cell culture produced a population in which 50,000 times as many particles were required to infect rabbit skin as to infect the chorioallantoic membrane of the chick embryo. The recent success of Appleyard (1961) in extracting from elementary bodies the protein antigen which engenders the production of and combines with the neutralizing antibody offers a new approach to the study of the invasion of cells by pox virus. Since antibody can neutralize only free virus or virus superficially adsorbed to the host cell, the neutralizing antigen must be essential to adsorption and penetration. The neutralizing antigen is probably distinct from the protein destroyed in heat-treated particles capable of being reactivated, because they have no difficulty getting inside host cells. Thus there is good evidence for the specific participation of at least two viral proteins in the early stages of pox-virus growth.

A phenomenon which may be a direct consequence of the act of invasion is the toxic action of vaccinia virus on cells in culture (Bernkopf *et al.*, 1959; Brown *et al.*, 1959). When cells are infected with high doses, so that each cell receives many virus particles, characteristic cytopathic effects ensue, and most of the cells die. The effect is so rapid as to make multiplication of the virus an unlikely explanation. Also, particles made non-infectious by ultraviolet irradiation are equally effective in producing the toxic effect, and metabolic inhibitors which prevent virus multiplication fail to prevent toxicity. It is probable that the simultaneous adsorption and penetration of a large number of elementary bodies is in itself toxic to the cell. Brown *et al.* (1959) have suggested a rough analogy to the bacteriophage-induced lysis-from-without of bacteria infected with high doses of virus (Delbrück, 1940). It seems unlikely that this toxic action in cell culture has any direct relation to toxic reactions in intact animals, chiefly because of the high ratio of virus to cell required for the effect, but it may offer possibilities for investigating the nature of the initial interaction between pox virus and cell.

Multiplication and Release

Why pox-virus multiplication kills the cell in which it occurs cannot yet be explained in chemical terms. As discussed in the preceding section, nuclear function, as shown by synthesis of DNA and cell division, proceeds for many hours after infection. However, the simultaneous initiation of DNA and antigen production at all synthetic sites in a multiply infected cell shows that some generalized change has occurred throughout the cytoplasm, and this presents the possibility of some sort of irreversible damage.

With respect to release, we have the problem of explaining how viruses which spread so readily from cell to cell in intact hosts and from host to host are released so poorly in experimental systems.

Hemagglutinin

When pox viruses grow in host cells, they produce a hemagglutinin for fowl erythrocytes (Nagler, 1942; North, 1944; Burnet and Stone, 1946). The hemagglutinin is distinct from the elementary body and is associated with particles about 65 mμ in diameter (Chu, 1948). Gillen *et al.* (1950) have shown that two distinct kinds of hemagglutinating particles are formed. The hemagglutinating activity is destroyed by lecithinases, showing that phospholipid is the active agglutinating moiety. Hemagglutination is inhibited by specific antibodies formed in infected animals, but the hemagglutinin is antigenically distinct from any antigen of the elementary body. The role of the hemagglutinin in pox-virus infections is unknown. It is probably not essential because some strains of virus do not form detectable amounts of hemagglutinin.

SOME REFLECTIONS ON THE PATTERN OF
POX-VIRUS MULTIPLICATION

The pox viruses differ in many important respects from the other obligate intracellular parasites that we have discussed.

They pass through a period of eclipse, they do not reproduce by fission, they contain only DNA and not RNA, they are not susceptible to chemotherapeutic agents, and they have no clearly demonstrated enzyme activities. In brief, the pox viruses behave as viruses are expected to behave (Lwoff, 1957, 1959). Their multiplication may be described in terms of the conventional picture of virus reproduction. The elementary body enters the cell and loses its identity when it is stripped of its protein coat. The liberated viral DNA then replaces host nucleic acid as a supplier of patterns for biosynthetic activity, and viral DNA and protein are synthesized. Finally, the viral subunits are assembled into a new generation of infectious virus.

Such a description offers a plausible explanation for the differences between a pox virus and a rickettsia or a member of the psittacosis group. However, the pox viruses have other properties which cannot so easily be fitted into the framework of a conventional viral reproductive mechanism.

One of these has to do with the size and complexity of the infective unit which is supposedly assembled from separately synthesized subunits. This problem may be approached by comparing the nucleic acid and protein content of vaccinia virus with that of viruses for which eclipse, separate synthesis of subunits, and final assembly constitute a generally accepted mode of reproduction. This has been done in Table V-1. We see that vaccinia virus has 10 times the mass of either influenza virus or bacteriophage T2 and 500 times the mass of poliovirus. Only in the amount of DNA in bacteriophage T2 do any of the values for the other viruses approach the corresponding one for vaccinia virus. However, the protein complement of T2, although one-twentieth the mass, has more known separate components than the vaccinial protein. The comparison is somewhat inconclusive. The pox viruses are definitely much larger than the other viruses in Table

V-1, but they are not of such a completely different order of magnitude as to rule out a common mode of multiplication. The non-genetic reactivation of heat-inactivated pox viruses points to an active and specific role for at least one protein in the initiation of infection. This is, of course, at variance with a simple viral theory of multiplication which ascribes only a passive protective role to the viral proteins. The presence of copper and flavinadenine dinucleotide in elementary

TABLE V-1*

NUCLEIC ACID AND PROTEIN CONTENT OF REPRESENTATIVE VIRUSES

	VIRUS			
	Polio	Influenza A	Bacterio-phage T2	Vaccinia
Dry weight of 1 particle (gm.)....	1×10^{-17}	5×10^{-16}	5×10^{-16}	5×10^{-15}
Particle weight................	6×10^{6}	3×10^{8}	3×10^{8}	3×10^{9}
Nucleic acid				
RNA (per cent).............	30	1	....	....
DNA (per cent).............	....	....	50	6
"Molecular weight" of nucleic acid per particle.................	2×10^{6}	3×10^{6}	1.5×10^{8}	2×10^{8}
Protein (per cent)..............	70	70	50	90
"Molecular weight" of protein per particle....................	4×10^{6}	2×10^{8}	1.5×10^{8}	3×10^{9}
Minimum number of distinct proteins......................	1	2	7	5

* Values are rounded off for ease of comparison. Data on animal viruses are from Shäfer (1959); data on bacteriophage T2 are mainly from Evans (1959).

bodies of vaccinia remains just as much an enigma today as when they were discovered there over 20 years ago. The only thing more difficult to explain than their function in vaccinial reproduction is why they are present if they are, indeed, without function. Finally, as pointed out earlier, the maturation of a developmental body into an elementary body must involve extensive rearrangement of the internal structure of the infective unit after it has been assembled from its subunits—an occurrence not accounted for by usual theories of virus multiplication.

However, none of these complicating factors offers any hint of an alternative non-viral mode of reproduction. They merely call attention to the complexity of the pox viruses and of the processes which give rise to them. There seems to be no unbridgeable gap in size and complexity between the large bacterial viruses and the pox viruses, and it is reasonable to assume for them a viral mechanism of reproduction more complicated than that of the other animal viruses and comparable only to that of the large phages.

This assumption implies a new cause for obligate intracellular parasitism—dependency on the host for synthetic enzymes. Here there does seem to be an unbridgeable gap—between a dependency on substrates, no matter how complex, and a dependency on enzymes. Whether this gap is real and indicative of an evolutionary hiatus or only apparent and indicative of lack of information can be decided only by more work.

REFERENCES

ADAMS, M. H. 1959. Bacteriophages. New York: Interscience Publishers, Inc.

ALLISON, A. C., and PERKINS, H. R. 1960. Nature, 188:796–98.

ANDRES, K. H., LIESKE, H., LIPPETT, H., MANNWEILER, E., NIELSEN, G., PETERS, D., and SEELEMAN, K. 1958. Deutsch. med. Wchnschr., 83: 1–21.

APPLEYARD, G. 1961. Nature, 190:465–66.

BANG, F. B. 1950. Bull. Johns Hopkins Hosp., 87:511–19.

BERNKOPF, H., NISHMI, M., and ROSIN, I. 1959. J. Immunol., 83:635–39.

BERRY, G. P., and DEDRICK, H. M. 1936. J. Bact., 31:50–51.

BLAND, J. O. W., and ROBINOW, C. F. 1939. J. Path. Bact., 48:381–403.

BRENNER, S., JACOB, F., and MESELSON, M. 1961. Nature, 190:576–81.

BROWN, A., MAYYASI, S. A., and OFFICER, J. E. 1959. J. Infect. Dis., 104: 193–202.

BURNET, F. M. 1936. Spec. Rept. Ser. M. Res. Comm. London, No. 220.

BURNET, F. M., and STONE, J. D. 1946. Australian J. Exper. Biol. M. Sc., 24:1–8.

CAIRNS, J. 1960. Virology, 11:603–23.

CHU, C. M. 1948. J. Hyg., 46:42–48.

The Pox Viruses

CRAIGIE, J. 1932. Brit. J. Exper. Path., 13:259–68.

CRAIGIE, J., and WISHART, F. O. 1934. Brit. J. Exper. Path., 15:390–98.

DAWSON, I. M., and McFARLANE, A. S. 1948. Nature, 161:464–66.

DELBRÜCK, M. 1940. J. Gen. Physiol., 23:643–60.

DULBECCO, R. 1952. Proc. Nat. Acad. Sc. U.S., 38:747–52.

EASTERBROOK, K. B. 1961. Virology, 15:404–16.

EPSTEIN, M. A. 1958. Brit. J. Exper. Path., 39:436–46.

EVANS, E. A., JR. 1959. In: The viruses, ed. F. M. BURNET and W. M. STANLEY, 3:459–74. New York: Academic Press, Inc.

FENNER, F. 1948. J. Path. Bact., 60:529–52.

———. 1949. J. Immunol., 63:341–73.

———. 1959. Virology, 8:499–507.

FENNER, F., and BURNET, F. M. 1957. Virology, 4:305–14.

FENNER, F., and COMBEN, B. M. 1958. Virology, 5:530–48.

FENNER, F., HOLMES, I. H., JOKLIK, W. K., and WOODROOFE, G. W. 1959. Nature, 183:1340–41.

FENNER, F., and WOODROOFE, G. M. 1960. Virology, 11:185–201.

FIRKET, H., and VERLY, W. G. 1958. Nature, 181:274–75.

FLEWETT, T. H. 1956. J. Hyg., 54:393–400.

FURNESS, G., and YOUNGNER, J. S. 1959. Virology, 9:386–95.

GAYLORD, W. H., and MELNICK, J. L. 1953. J. Exper. Med., 98:157–72.

GEMMEL, A., and CAIRNS, J. 1959. Virology, 8:381–83.

GEMMEL, A., and FENNER, F. 1960. Virology, 11:219–35.

GESSLER, A. E., BENDER, C. E., and PARKINSON, M. C. 1956. Trans. N.Y. Acad. Sc., 18:701–3.

GILLEN, A., BURR, M. M., and NAGLER, F. P. 1950. J. Immunol., 65:701–6.

GREEN, R. H., ANDERSON, T. F., and SMADEL, J. E. 1942. J. Exper. Med., 75:651–56.

GROS, H., HIATT, H., GILBERT, W., KURLAND, C. G., RISEBROUGH, R. W., and WATSON, J. D. 1961. Nature, 190:581–85.

GUTHRIE, G. D., and SINSHEIMER, R. L. 1960. J. Mol. Biol., 2:297–305.

HAMPARIAN, V. V., MÜLLER, V., and HUMMELER, K. 1958. J. Immunol., 80:468–75.

HANAFUSA, T., HANAFUSA, H., and KAMAHORA, J. 1959. Virology, 8:525–27.

HIGASHI, N. 1959. In: Progress in medical virology, ed. E. BERGER and J. L. MELNICK, 2:43–72. New York: Hafner Publishing Co.

HIGASHI, N., OZAKI, Y., and ICHIMIYA, M. 1960. J. Ultrastructure Res., 3:270–81.

HOAGLAND, C. L., LAVIN, G. I., SMADEL, J. E., and RIVERS, T. M. 1940. J. Exper. Med., 72:139–47.

HOAGLAND, C. L., SMADEL, J. E., and RIVERS, T. M. 1940. J. Exper. Med., 71:737–50.

160

References

HOAGLAND, C. L., WARD, S. M., SMADEL, J.E., and RIVERS, T. M. 1940. Proc. Soc. Exper. Biol. Med., 45:669–71.

HOAGLAND, C. L., WARD, S. M., SMADEL, J. E., and RIVERS, T. M. 1941a. J. Exper. Med., 74:69–80.

———. 1941b. Ibid., pp. 133–44.

———. 1942. Ibid., 76:163–73.

HOLT, S. J., and EPSTEIN, M. A. 1958. Brit. J. Exper. Path., 39:472–79.

HORSFALL, F. L., JR. 1959. In: The viruses, ed. F. M. BURNET and W. M. STANLEY, 3:195–224. New York: Academic Press, Inc.

ISAACS, A. 1959. In: The viruses, ed. F. M. BURNET and W. H. STANLEY, 3:111–56. New York: Academic Press, Inc.

JACOB, F., and MONOD, J. 1961. J. Mol. Biol., 3:318–56.

JOKLIK, W. K. 1959. Virology, 9:417–24.

JOKLIK, W. K., ABEL, P., and HOLMES, I. H. 1960. Nature, 186:992–93.

JOKLIK, W. K., HOLMES, I. H., and BRIGGS, M. J. 1960. Virology, 11:202–18.

JOKLIK, W. K., and RODRICK, J. McN. 1959. Virology, 9:396–416.

JOKLIK, W. K., WOODROOFE, G. W., HOLMES, I. H., and FENNER, F. 1960. Virology, 11:168–84.

KAPLAN, C., and VALENTINE, R. C. 1959. J. Gen. Microbiol., 20:612–19.

KILHAM, L. 1957. Proc. Soc. Exper. Biol. Med., 95:57–62.

LEDINGHAM, J. C. G. 1931. Lancet, 221:525–26.

LOH, P. C., and RIGGS, J. L. 1961. J. Exper. Med., 114:149–60.

LWOFF, A. 1957. J. Gen. Microbiol., 17:239–53.

———. 1959. In: The viruses, ed. F. M. BURNET and W. M. STANLEY, 3:187–201. New York: Academic Press, Inc.

LYNEN, F., KNAPPE, J., LORCH, E., JUTTING, G., and RENGELMANN, E. 1959. Angew. Chem., 71:481–86.

McFARLANE, A. S. 1940. Trans. Faraday Soc., 36:257–64.

McFARLANE, A. S., and MACFARLANE, M. G. 1939. Nature, 144:376–77.

McFARLANE, A. S., MACFARLANE, M. G., AMIES, C. R., and EAGLES, G. H. 1939. Brit. J. Exper. Path., 20:485–501.

MACFARLANE, M. G., and DOLBY, D. E. 1940. Brit. J. Exper. Path., 21:219–27.

MACFARLANE, M. G., and SALAMAN, M. H. 1938. Brit. J. Exper. Path., 19:184–91.

MAGEE, W. E., SHEEK, M. R., and BURROUS, M. J. 1960. Virology, 11:296–99.

MAGEE, W. E., SHEEK, M. R., and SAGIK, B. P. 1959. Fed. Proc., 18:582.

MEYER, F., MACKAL, R. P., TAO, M., and EVANS, E. A., JR. 1961. J. Biol. Chem., 236:1141–43.

MORGAN, C., ELLISON, S. A., ROSE, H. M., and MOORE, D. H. 1954. J. Exper. Med., 100:301–10.

———. 1955. Exper. Cell Res., 9:572–78.

MORGAN, C., and WYKOFF, R. W. G. 1950. J. Immunol., 65:285–95.

NAGLER, F. P. O. 1942. M. J. Australia, 1:281–83.

NISHIMURA, C., and TAGAYA, I. 1959. Jap. J. M. Sc. Biol., 12:405–20.

NORTH, E. A. 1944. Australian J. Exper. Biol. Med. Sc., 22:105–9.

NOYES, W. F., and WATSON, B. 1955. J. Exper. Med., 102:237–42.

OCHOA, S., and KAZIRO, Y. 1961. Fed. Proc., 20:982–88.

OFFICER, J. E., and BROWN, A. 1960. J. Infect. Dis., 107:283–99.

———. 1961. Virology, 14:88–99.

OVERMAN, J. R., and SHARP, D. G. 1959. J. Exper. Med., 110:461–80.

PARKER, R. F., BRONSON, L. H., and GREEN, R. H. 1941. J. Exper. Med., 74:263–81.

PETERS, D. 1956. Nature, 178:1453–55.

———. 1959. Zentralbl. Bakt. (orig.), 176:259–94.

———. 1960. Proc. IV Internat. Conf. Electron Microscopy (Berlin, 1958), 2:554–73.

PETERS, D., and STOECKENIUS, W. 1954. Ztschr. Naturforsch., 9b:524–29.

PFAU, C. J., and McCREA, J. F. 1961. Bact. Proc., p. 148.

PICKELS, E. G., and SMADEL, J. E. 1938. J. Exper. Med., 68:583–606.

POSTLETHWAITE, R., and MAITLAND, H. B. 1960. J. Hyg., 58:133–45.

RANDALL, C. C., and GAFFORD, L. G. 1961. Bact. Proc., p. 148.

SALZMAN, N. P. 1960. Virology, 10:150–52.

SCHUSTER, H. 1960. *In:* The nucleic acids, ed. E. CHARGAFF and J. N. DAVIDSON, 3:245–303. New York: Academic Press, Inc.

SHACK, J., and KILHAM, L. 1959. Proc. Soc. Exper. Biol. Med., 100:726–29.

SHÄFER, W. 1959. *In:* The viruses, ed. F. M. BURNET and W. M. STANLEY, 1:475–504. New York: Academic Press, Inc.

SHEDLOVSKY, T., and SMADEL, J. E. 1940. J. Exper. Med., 72:511–21.

SHEEK, M. R. 1961. Doctoral dissertation, University of Illinois, Urbana.

SHEEK, M. R., and MAGEE, W. E. 1961. Virology, 15:146–63.

SMADEL, J. E., and HOAGLAND, C. L. 1942. Bact. Rev., 6:79–110.

SMADEL, J. E., LAVIN, G. I., and DUBOS, R. J. 1940. J. Exper. Med., 71:373–89.

SMADEL, J. E., PICKELS, E. G., and SHEDLOVSKY, T. 1938. J. Exper. Med., 68:607–27.

SMADEL, J. E., RIVERS, T. M., and PICKELS, E. G. 1939. J. Exper. Med., 70:379–85.

STAEHELIN, M. 1959. *In:* Progress in medical virology, ed. E. BERGER and J. L. MELNICK, 2:1–42. New York: Hafner Publishing Co. Inc.

TAMM, I., and BABLANIAN, R. 1960. J. Exper. Med., 11:351–68.

WOODROOFE, G. W., and FENNER, F. 1960. Virology, 12:272–82.

WOODRUFF, A. M., and GOODPASTURE, E. W. 1931. Am. J. Path., 7:209–22.

WYATT, G. R., and COHEN, S. S. 1953. Biochem. J., 55:774–82.

WYKOFF, R. W. G. 1951. Proc. Nat. Acad. Sc. U.S., 37:565–69.

YAMAMOTO, T., and BLACK, F. L. 1961. Bact. Proc., p. 147.

CHAPTER VI

In Search of an Evolutionary History

The examples of obligate intracellular parasitism that we have just examined range in complexity from the clearly non-viral to the just-barely viral; hence it is appropriate to ask ourselves whether our present knowledge of these agents gives any hint of an orderly evolutionary progression from free-living micro-organisms to viruses. Before attempting to answer this general question, let us ask a more restricted one: Are there obvious evolutionary relationships among the four groups of obligate intracellular parasites that have been the subjects of this book?

It is at once apparent that the plasmodia stand alone within the group of four. They are recognizably kin only to other members of the class Sporozoa, whose origin is a puzzle to protozoölogists. The Sporozoa must have evolved from free-living Protozoa in ancient times, so ancient that none of the descendants of their free-living ancestors have survived to the present. It looks as if the adoption of an intracellular mode of life permitted the very successful survival of a whole class of Protozoa that would otherwise have perished.

This leaves us with the rickettsiae, the psittacosis group, and the pox viruses. It would be so satisfying and exciting to find signs of direct and immediate kinship among these great groups of intracellular parasites that it is disappointing to find that they are not there. There are many resemblances between the rickettsiae and the psittacosis group, but they are all general ones and may be accounted for by the obvious bacterial heritage of both. There are no peculiar common properties indicative of recent divergence from a common stock. Other properties, such as the almost invariable arthropod vectors in rickettsial diseases and the complete absence of such vectors in diseases caused by the psittacosis group, are positive arguments against a recent common origin. Nothing about the pox viruses provides as close a link to the bacteria as the presence of muramic acid or the susceptibility to antibacterial agents does for the rickettsiae and the psittacosis group. It might be argued that the pox group has evolved so far from a bacterial starting point that all distinctive bacterial characters have been lost, but opinions about the origin of the pox group are really a matter of faith and not of information.

So, to answer our question about evolutionary relationships among the restricted group we have chosen to analyze in detail, there is no evidence that any one of the four is in the direct line of descent of any of the others; the rickettsiae and the psittacosis group are remotely related by virtue of a distant bacterial origin; and the malarial parasites and the pox viruses are so unlike any of the other agents that a valid comparison is impossible.

Granting that these agents all represent the present-day culmination of long-independent lines of evolution, have we learned anything about patterns of parasitic specialization from this exhaustive consideration of their biochemical properties? The principle generally invoked to explain the development of obligate intracellular parasitism is that of degenerative or regressive evolution, first clearly stated by Green (1935) and Laidlaw (1938).[1] It is unfortunate that the terms "regressive" and "degenerative" have been applied here. However they may have evolved, the plasmodia, the rickett-

[1] For a recent stimulating application of this concept to the origin of viruses see Burnet (1960).

siae, the psittacosis group, and the pox viruses are highly successful organisms, well adapted to their environments, widely distributed throughout the biosphere, and in absolutely no danger of extinction. There is no reason at all to consider them as imperfect or degenerate organisms or to imply that the evolutionary mechanisms responsible for their development are in any way unusual.

Let us abandon the malarial parsites as lost to our discussion, assume that the rickettsiae, the psittacosis group, and the pox viruses are all of ultimate bacterial origin, and add to this group, for the sake of comparison, a facultatively intracellular bacterium. The most suitable species for this purpose is the causative agent of tularemia, *Pasteurella tularensis*. It is the same size as rickettsiae, can grow intracellularly, is transmitted by insect vectors, and is cultured only with difficulty in complex artificial media.

We have already minimally defined a virus as a particle with a protective protein coat surrounding a nucleic acid core which is capable of causing the replication of the entire particle within a host cell. We now need a similar minimum definition of a bacterium. Since a bacterium is more complicated than a virus, its definition will likewise be more complicated. On a gross morphological level, a bacterium must possess a rigid cell wall to give it mechanical strength, a cell membrane to regulate the flow of metabolites in and out of the cell, a cytoplasm to contain the energy-yielding and biosynthetic enzyme units, and a nuclear body to contain the genetic apparatus. On a molecular level, the bacterium must contain DNA, RNA, protein, polysaccharide, lipid, and low-molecular-weight coenzymes and substrates. Functionally, the bacterium takes in simple substrates from the medium and oxidizes a portion of them to generate metabolically useful energy, with which it converts other simple substances into its own specific macromolecules of DNA, RNA, and protein, employing for this purpose enzyme proteins synthesized under the immediate control of RNA molecules whose specificity is in turn determined by the nuclear DNA. When sufficient new cell material is formed, the bacterium divides in such a way that each daughter cell receives a full complement of DNA.

It is a long way from *P. tularensis* to vaccinia virus. What we must ask ourselves now is whether the rickettsiae and the psittacosis group provide reasonable examples of what intermediate stages in such an evolution might have been or whether there are large discontinuities in the hypothetical pathway from bacterium to virus.

Rickettsiae are clearly small bacteria, and the most striking difference between them and *P. tularensis* is that they cannot be grown on artificial media, while the tularemia agent can. This inability seems to stem from two main causes. First, rickettsiae exhibit a highly restricted range of enzymatic activities, even when compared with the comparatively incompetent *P. tularensis*. The loss of the glycolytic cycle without substitution of any alternative mode of glucose breakdown is particularly striking. Second, they seem to show some impairment in controlling the flow of low-molecular-weight substances in and out of the cell. Although such changes may logically be expected in the course of adaptation to an intracellular environment, the rickettsiae do not appear to have traveled far enough along the road from bacterium to virus to be of much help in mapping the way.

The psittacosis group has traveled farther. If, as suggested in chapter iv, they have lost their energy-producing systems and depend on their hosts to generate energy-rich compounds for them to use in their biosynthetic reactions, this represents a major difference between the psittacosis group and bacteria and is one which would have to evolve in going from bacterium to virus. Such an energy dependency would also necessitate a change in the permeability of the cell membrane, because most energy-rich compounds do not pass freely into ordinary intact cells. A unique characteristic of the psittacosis group and one that well may be of evolutionary significance is their growth cycle, with its alternation of particle types: a multiplying, weakly infectious one and a nonmultiplying, highly infectious one. This growth cycle may be taken as a foreshadowing of the viral reproductive mechanism in which the multiplying form is free nucleic acid and the non-multiplying, highly infectious form is the nucleic acid incased in a protein coat.

We must take a big jump from psittacosis to pox because there is no convenient steppingstone between. The distinctive bacterial cell wall, still possessed by the rickettsiae and the psittacosis group, is almost certainly absent in the pox viruses. Chemical analyses on the empty membranes left after pepsin-DNase-pepsin digestion are unfortunately not available, but, even without these data, there is good evidence that the empty membranes are not cell-wall analogues. First, the insusceptibility of the pox viruses to antibiotics is indicative of a lack of a bacteria-like cell wall and cell membrane. Penicillin has been shown, beyond all reasonable doubt, to inhibit cell-wall synthesis at the cell membrane, and there is evidence of a somewhat less comprehensive nature that the site of action of almost all antibiotics on bacteria is the cell membrane (reviewed by Landman, 1962). Second, the susceptibility of pox-virus particles to attack by pepsin and papain and their resistance to lipid solvents is just exactly opposite to that expected of a particle with an outer covering similar to a bacterial cell wall.

The second large difference between pox particles and psittacosis particles is the absence of RNA in the pox viruses. There is little chance of there being any RNA in the mature elementary bodies, which have been the subject of exhaustive

167

chemical analysis. It is possible that the immature developmental bodies may contain RNA, but there is at present only the possibility and no evidence. If we assume the absence of RNA, then we are, of necessity, also assuming a viral mode of reproduction, because all current theories of protein synthesis require the participation of RNA. Without RNA, there is no protein synthesis, and, without protein synthesis, an organismal type of reproduction of new individuals from existing individuals is not possible.

It is this step from an organism with the DNA-RNA-protein relationship typical of cells in general to one in which the chain has been broken by the insertion of the RNA of the host that is so hard to visualize and for which no intermediate steps can be found. It is also potentially the most interesting one. In the face of such an appalling lack of information, speculation would be rash indeed, and we are forced to conclude this search for an evolutionary history of obligate intracellular parasitism on a rather flat note of exhortation to study the familiar intracellular parasites with greater diligence and thoroughness and to examine a much greater number of the lesser known ones. We can hope that, in the resulting greater depth of information about a wider variety of obligate intracellular parasites, we may be able to see patterns of development and interrelationships that are now completely obscure.

REFERENCES

BURNET, F. M. 1960. Principles of animal virology, chap. xix. 2d ed. New York: Academic Press, Inc.

GREEN, R. G. 1935. Science, **82**:443–45.

LAIDLAW, P. P. 1938. Virus diseases and viruses. London: Cambridge University Press.

LANDMAN, O. 1962. Ann. N.Y. Acad. Sc., in press.

Index